Fabíola Silva Garcia Praça

Release and Permeation of Transdermal Products

Fabíola Silva Garcia Praça

Release and Permeation of Transdermal Products

In vitro release and permeation of transdermal products: a methodological study of experimental apparatus and conditions

ScienciaScripts

Imprint

Cover image: www.ingimage.com

This book is a translation from the original published under ISBN 978-3-330-76977-9.

Publisher:
Sciencia Scripts
is a trademark of
Dodo Books Indian Ocean Ltd. and OmniScriptum S.R.L publishing group

120 High Road, East Finchley, London, N2 9ED, United Kingdom
Str. Armeneasca 28/1, office 1, Chisinau MD-2012, Republic of Moldova, Europe
Managing Directors: Ieva Konstantinova, Victoria Ursu
info@omniscriptum.com

Printed at: see last page
ISBN: 978-620-8-62677-8

SUMMARY

DEDICATION

I dedicate the completion of this work to what I value most, my family.

.. to my father, who has always guided me along the path of knowledge with great love and affection, teaching me to have security, confidence and perseverance in the pursuit of my goals...

...my mother who, with great dedication, taught me to be a daughter, a woman, a wife and a professional...

.. to my sisters for sharing their greatest achievements with me and welcoming me in the most difficult moments of this process called life....

....e to my husband for turning simple moments into unforgettable ones

ACKNOWLEDGMENTS

To my advisor Prof. Dr. Dr. Maria Vitória Lopes Badra Bentley for the opportunity, guidance, trust and friendship

To all my colleagues in the Pharmacotechnics and Pharmaceutical Technology laboratory of the Department of Pharmaceutical Sciences at FCFRP-USP, for their encouragement and collaboration.

To José Orestes Del Ciampo and Henrique Diniz, employees of the Pharmacotechnics and Pharmaceutical Technology laboratory of the Department of Pharmaceutical Sciences at FCFRP-USP, for their companionship.

To Dr. Fabiana Testa Moura Vicentini and Profª. Eliane Candiani Arantes, for their valuable contributions during the qualifying exam for my doctoral thesis.

To the professors and staff of the postgraduate program at FCFRP-USP, who contributed to my education with great professionalism.

The São Paulo State Research Foundation - FAPESP

To the National Council for Scientific and Technological Development - CNPq

To all those who, directly or indirectly, helped make this work possible.

"Speak to their hearts"

Nelson Mandela

SUMMARY

PRAÇA, FABIOLA SILVA GARCIA. ***In vitro* release and permeation of transdermal products: a methodological study of apparatus and experimental conditions.**

Transdermal drug release has several therapeutic advantages over oral or parenteral administration. To date, there is no method in the Brazilian Pharmacopoeia for carrying out drug release tests on transdermal patches. Other official compendia, such as the American, British and European Pharmacopoeia, describe the powder-on-disc apparatus, the rotating cylinder and the reciprocal support. Currently, the literature describes various types of diffusion cells for transdermal release, of which the Franz diffusion cell has been the most widely used for both transdermal patches and semi-solid forms and has been used in pharmacotechnical development, biopharmaceutical characterization and quality control. The aim of this study was to establish criteria for the most appropriate choice of equipment and *in vitro* methodologies for evaluating the transdermal release of drugs, using nicotine as a model drug. To this end, *in vitro* skin release and retention tests were used and compared with each other using the powder-on-disk method and the modified Franz diffusion cell method in a static and continuous flow system. The validation of the factors that influence the *in vitro* release rate of nicotine was fundamental to the choice of the receptor medium, the choice of the stirring speed that promoted the most similarity in the release profile in different equipment as well as the choice of the most suitable biological membrane for the proposed method. The release results, both in terms of the amount of nicotine released and its flow, showed similarity when using different equipment, indicating possible interchangeability between the proposed methods for transdermal nicotine release. *In vitro* skin permeation tests in a Franz vertical diffusion cell showed no significant differences in the different biological membrane models used, which were pig ear skin, hairless mouse skin and rattlesnake skin hydrated for 24 hours. The amount of nicotine permeated in up to 8 hours, as well as the permeation flux were significantly lower for the FDA method when compared to the results obtained using the Franz vertical diffusion cell in both static and continuous flow systems. These results may be related to the physical structure of the Franz vertical diffusion cell equipment, since it offers an occlusive system, making it difficult for the adhesive to come into contact with the receiving medium. In this way, the results of this project may indicate the use of the Franz vertical diffusion cell for *in vitro* tests on the release and skin permeation of nicotine in transdermal pharmaceutical forms, and may be applied to research into formulation development, quality control and pharmaceutical equivalence tests for generic products. The results of this research are an important tool for discussions on pharmaceutical equivalence tests and quality control of transdermal drugs, as well as understanding possible process errors. They could also provide data for the indication of protocols for the Brazilian Pharmacopoeia and scientific research into transdermal drug delivery systems.

Keywords: *in vitro* release and permeation; transdermal systems, nicotine, intra-laboratory validation.

1. LITERATURE REVIEW

1.1 THE SKIN

The skin is the outer covering of the body, considered the largest and heaviest organ in the human body, and is practically identical in all human ethnic groups. In dark-skinned individuals, melanocytes produce more melanin than in light-skinned individuals, but their number is similar (**Figure 1**). (BARRY, 1983)

It is subdivided into three distinct layers: the stratified and vascularized epidermis, the dermis and the subcutaneous hypodermis, as well as several attached organs, such as hair follicles, sweat glands and sebaceous glands (JUNQUEIRA *et al.*, 1995).

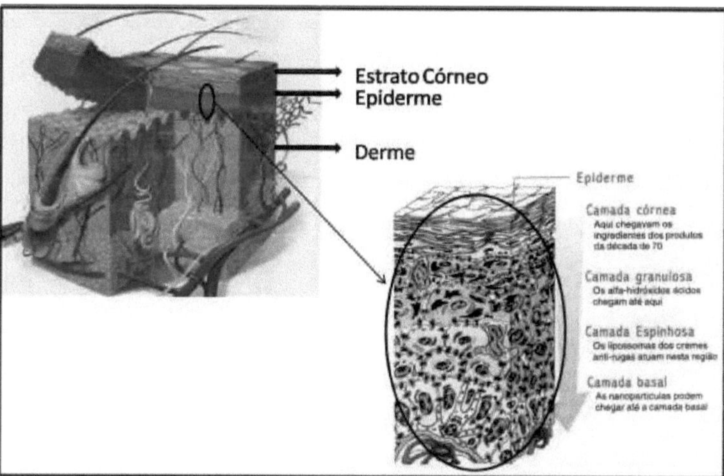

Figure 1 - Image of human skin and morphological subdivisions (stratum corneum, epidermis and dermis), reproduced from the book Piel Eudemica: Morfogia y Fisiologia (Lorenzo Pons Gimier).

The epidermis is made up of a keratinized stratified sidewalk epithelium (squamous cells in several layers) where the main cell is the keratinocyte (or keratinocyte), which produces keratin. There are also nests of melanocytes, which produce melanin, a brown pigment that absorbs ultraviolet (UV) rays; and immune cells, mainly giant Langerhans cells with membrane extensions (ABRAHAM *et al.,* 1995).

In skin permeation studies, the epidermis is the layer of skin that deserves the most attention. The epidermis can be subdivided into the basal layer, which is the deepest and comes into contact with the dermis; the spinous layer, made up of conical or flattened cells with more keratin than the basal cells, which begin to form cell junctions with each other, promoting the appearance of spines; the granular layer made up of flattened cells with prominent keratin granules and others such as extracellular substance and other proteins; the lucid layer made up of hyaline and eosinophilic flattened cells due to very numerous protein granules and the stratum corneum (BARRY, 1983).

The stratum corneum (SC) is one of the main barriers to drug penetration. It is made up of flattened eosinophilic cells without a nucleus with a large number of filaments, mainly keratins. The lipids in this matrix are organized in multilamellar structures, in which hydrophilic and lipophilic domains alternate, which can serve as a pathway for drug transport (BARRY, 1983; SINKO 2008).

The dermis is a connective tissue that supports the epidermis. It is made up of fibrillar elements such as collagen and elastin and other elements of the extracellular matrix such as structural proteins, glycosaminoglycans, ions and solvation water. It is subdivided into two layers: the papillary layer in contact with the epidermis, made up of loose connective tissue, and the reticular layer made up of dense, unshaped connective tissue, where collagen fibers predominate.

The dermis is where the blood and lymphatic vessels that vascularize the epidermis are located, as well as the nerves and sensory organs associated with them (GAO *et al.,* 1998).

The hypodermis is called adipose tissue that protects the body against the cold. It is a loose or adipose connective tissue that connects the dermis and the muscular fascia, and this layer of adipose tissue varies according to the person and location on the body (JUNQUEIRA *et al.,* 1995).

The skin is responsible for the functions of thermoregulation, defense, perception and protection of the human body, among others (ABRAHAM *et al.,* 1995).

The work of MICHAELS and collaborators (1975) on the possible routes of drug release culminated in the analogy of the skin to a wall composed of bricks, due to its barrier function and consequent limitations in penetration.

1.2 TRANSDERMAL RELEASE SYSTEMS

In the 1950s, a new concept of releasing drugs through the skin was introduced, but despite a growing advance in scientific research into this new discovery, it was only in 1979 that the first generation of skin-applied drugs for nausea, vomiting and angina associated with travel, especially sea travel, was approved by the Food and Drug Administration (FDA) and made commercially available in the United States (ALLEN *et al.,* 2007).

However, it was the commercialization of transdermal nicotine patches used in anti-smoking treatment that provided the necessary impetus for this transdermal drug delivery technology (ALLEN *et al.,* 2007).

Transdermal therapeutic systems (TTSs) facilitate the passage of therapeutic quantities of drugs through the skin, with the aim of reaching the bloodstream to exert systemic effects (ALLEN *et al.,* 2007).

The basic process involved in transdermal drug release technology is the percutaneous or transdermal absorption of the drug (SINKO, 2008). Not all substances have characteristics suitable for transdermal administration, due to their physical and chemical properties, including molecular mass, solubility, partition coefficient and dissociation constant (ALLEN *et al.,* 2007). One example is the diffusion of 15 polar drugs through the skin which occurs much faster through the viable skin tissue, Epidermis and Dermis (EP + D) when compared to the speed through the EC (ALLEN *et al.,* 2007).

The permeation flow of the drug through the stratum corneum is expressed through the mathematical model of Fick's law, shown in Equation 1 (HIGUCHI, 1960).

(Eq. 1)

$$J = \frac{D_M \, x \, C_{s.m}}{L} \, x \, \frac{C_V}{C_{s.m}}$$

where J is the flux; D_M is the diffusion coefficient of the drug through the membrane; Cs,m is the solubility of the drug in the membrane; L is the diffusion length of the drug through the membrane; Cv is the concentration of the drug dissolved in the vehicle and Cs,v is the solubility of the drug in the vehicle.

TTSs are designed to induce the drug to pass through all layers of the skin until it reaches the bloodstream. Technically, they are divided into two distinct classes: monolithic systems and membrane-controlled systems (ALLEN *et al.,* 2007).

Monolithic transdermal release systems have the drug incorporated into a matrix layer composed of a polymeric material which controls the release of the drug. This polymeric material is usually solubilized together with the drug to form the matrix and after going through the drying process, this mixture is incorporated between the front and back layers of the transdermal patch (ALLEN *et al.,* 2007).

Membrane-controlled systems contain a reservoir, usually in liquid or gel form, containing the drug, a membrane that controls the release rate and an adhesive layer. The advantage over monolithic systems is that the rate of release remains constant, since the amount of drug in the reservoir remains saturated. In general, TTSs are made up of different numbers of layers, including an outer layer which protects the system from the external environment and from losses, a matrix or reservoir layer which stores and releases the drug into the skin, an adhesive layer to keep the drug in contact with the skin and a final protective layer which must be removed before use (ALLEN *et al.,* 2007).

Allen *et al.* (2007) presented a table containing some examples of the structure and composition of various TTSs. For nicotine, four commercially available systems were demonstrated, Habitrol® , Nicoderm® , Nicotrol® and Prostep® . Habitrol® (*Novartis Consumer*) consists of an adhesive disk, aluminized outer layer, acrylate adhesive layer, nicotine solution in methacrylate acid copolymer, acrylate adhesive layer and disposable aluminium protective coating which covers the adhesive layer and must be removed before use. Nicoderm® *(Smitthkline Beecham Consumer*) consists of a rectangular adhesive, an occlusive outer layer of polyethylene, aluminum, polyester, ethylenevinyl acetate copolymer, a nicotine reservoir in a copolymer matrix, a polyethylene membrane to control the speed of release, a polysobylene adhesive layer and a protective coating that must be removed before application. Nicotrol® *(McNeil Consumer)* consists of a rectangular adhesive, an outer layer of laminated polyester film, an adhesive that controls the speed of release, nicotine and a disposable liner that must be removed before use. Finally, Prostep® (*Lederle*) is an adhesive disk made up of a beige foam strip, acrylate adhesive, gelatine outer sheet with polyethylene coating, nicotine gel matrix, protective foil and disposable liner that must be removed before use.

1.3 ADVANTAGES OF TRANSDERMAL drug DELIVERY SYSTEMS

The transdermal release of drugs has several therapeutic advantages when compared to oral or parenteral administration (KEMKEN *et al.,* 1991). Among the advantages of the systems are (ANSEL *et al.,* 2000):

J Avoid difficulties caused by gastrointestinal pH, enzymatic activity, drug interactions and interactions with food, drink and orally administered drugs.

J Substitute oral administration when this route is unsuitable, such as in cases of vomiting and/or diarrhea.

J Avoid the first-pass effect, i.e. the initial passage of the drug through the portal and systemic circulations after gastrointestinal absorption, thus avoiding its possible inactivation by hepatic and digestive enzymes.

J Avoid the risks and inconvenience of parenteral administration and the variable metabolism and absorption associated with oral administration.

J Provide several doses a day with a single application, thus increasing the patient's cooperation.

J Increase the activity of drugs with a short half-life, due to the system's reservoir and controlled release characteristics.

J Allow the rapid interruption of the effect of the drugs, if desired, with their removal.

J To allow quick and easy administration of medication in emergencies, for example in unconscious and comatose patients.

1.4 *in vitro* release of pharmaceuticals as a support for scientific research and quality control of transdermal products

The *in vitro* drug release test is a very important tool in the pharmaceutical industry, both in product development and in routine quality control. Although it was initially developed for solid pharmaceutical forms, this test has also been applied to non-solid pharmaceutical forms, such as suspensions, transdermal patches, suppositories and others (MARCOLONGO & STORPIRTIS, 2003).

In order to understand the *in vitro* release of drugs, some of the significant events involved in carrying out the test must be fully understood, including (GORDON 1997):

J The application of an infinite layer of the release system, i.e. the sample being an ointment, gel or cream, on the surface of the membrane between the sample and the receptor fluid.

J Evaporation of the vehicle when associated with changes in the drug's activity.

J Drug dissolution in the vehicle

J Drug partitioning in the membrane

J Diffusion of the drug through the skin membrane by the transepidermal route, in which the drug penetrates the stratum corneum, reaches the viable epidermis, reaches the dermis and capillaries and enters the bloodstream, or by the transfollicular route in which the drug penetrates the sebum and hair follicles until it reaches the dermis and capillaries and enters the bloodstream.

J Systemic drug clearance (*clearance*)

Drug release can be simply defined as the process by which a drug is released from its pharmaceutical form and becomes available for absorption by the body (CHOWDARY *et al.*, 1987).

In vitro release tests are relevant in quality control and at different stages of a drug's life cycle. In the early stages of pharmacotechnical development, they are useful for identifying critical variables in production, choosing between different formulations, optimizing them and carrying out risk assessments, as in the case of modified release pharmaceutical forms.

During the production phase, *in vitro* release tests are important for batch release and stability testing, since the release characteristics of a product must remain constant throughout its shelf life and are also very useful for assessing the impact that certain changes, such as the use of different equipment or a change of manufacturing site, may have on the final product (ABUZARUR *et al.,* 1997; MANADAS *et al.,* 2002 and BRASIL, 2003).

With the advancement of technology, drug release research, the modernization of testing and more emphasis on the predictability of therapeutic effects, drug release testing has become increasingly popular. One of the oldest scientific articles on dissolution was published in 1897 and is entitled "The Rate of Solubility of Solid Substances in Their Own Solutions". The authors realized the importance of the subject and carried out experiments which led them to conclude that the rate of solubilization, according to the diffusion law, would be proportional to the concentration of the saturated solution film formed in the diffusion layer (NOYES *et al.,* 1897).

According to WAGNER (1971), between 1900 and 1903, Brunner and Toloczko showed that the proportionality constant of the Noyes-Whitney equation is dependent on the area and structure of the exposed surface, the intensity of agitation or flow, the temperature and the experimental apparatus (WAGNER, 1971).

In 1904, Nernst used Fick's diffusion law to establish a new relationship between the proportionality constant and the diffusion coefficient of the solute, allowing the thickness of the diffusion layer to be estimated. Based on this, ideas were put forward that all heterogeneous reactions depend on the rate of diffusion of the solute/solution equilibrium film that forms immediately at the interface (NERNST, 1904; WAGNER, 1971; ABDOU *et al.,* 1989 and BANAKAR 1992).

However, Klein was the first researcher to determine the dissolution rate of a tablet in 1932. A year later, Elliott, using Klein's apparatus, published graphs showing the amount of drug dissolved as a function of time from tablets containing five different drugs (WAGNER, 1971).

Until the early 1950s, experiments involving drug release were focused on the physicochemical characteristics of the drug, not necessarily including the pharmaceutical forms that contained them. From then on, the focus of experimentation shifted to evaluating the effects of drug release on the biological activity of the product. In the 1960s, the first apparatus for carrying out release tests on solid pharmaceutical forms was described (WAGNER, 1971).

1.4.1 Apparatus for in vitro release tests of topical and transdermal preparations

In 1970, the American Pharmacopoeia (Edition XVIII) published the first dissolution test and in 1975 (Edition XIX) it recommended two release apparatuses for solid pharmaceutical forms, Apparatus 1 (basket) and Apparatus 2 (feet), which are still the most widely used apparatuses today. As new drugs and drug release systems were studied, interest in drug release studies intensified (WAGNER, 1971). In 1990, the American Pharmacopoeia (Edition XXII) incorporated three apparatuses for the release of transdermal pharmaceutical forms: foot-on-disk apparatus, rotating cylinder apparatus and reciprocating cylinder support apparatus (**Figure 2**).

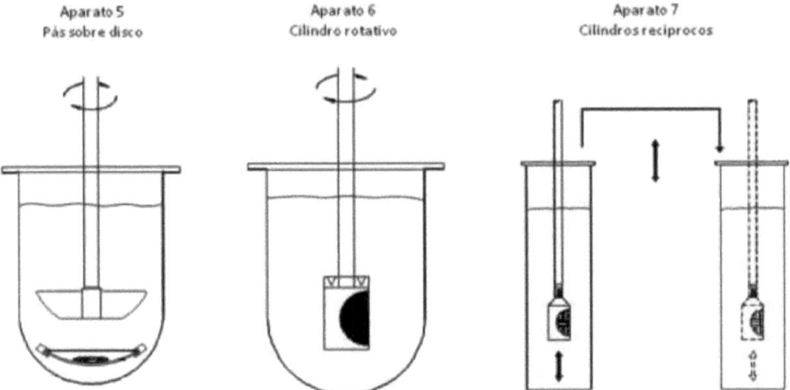

Figura 2. Schematic demonstration of apparatus 5, 6 and 7 described in the American Pharmacopoeia - USP 29).

The pad-on-disk apparatus described as Apparatus 5 in the American Pharmacopoeia is currently also described in the British and European Pharmacopoeia and recommended as a release method for transdermals by the FDA (Shah *et al.*, 1988). It should be used with the sink apparatus and a stainless steel disk to fix the transdermal system to the bottom of the tank. The disk should keep the transdermal system stretched parallel to the spatula, with the drug release surface facing upwards. The pH of the dissolution medium should be between 5.0 and 6.0 to reflect skin conditions, the same reason for using a temperature of 32°C (± 0.5) and the agitation considered appropriate is around 50 to 100 rpm (SIEWERT *et al.,* 2003).

Another device is the rotating cylinder, considered device 6 by the American Pharmacopoeia and also provided for by the British and European Pharmacopoeia, in which the rod with the handle is replaced by a rotating cylinder in which the pharmaceutical form is placed on the outside. (USP 29, 2006)

The third apparatus provided for by the American Pharmacopoeia is the reciprocating support, which uses a system similar to that of reciprocating cylinders with modifications for placing transdermal systems (USP 29). The conditions suggested for apparatus 6 and 7 are the same as for apparatus 5 (FDA) (SIEWERT *et al.,* 2003).

The evolution in the number of monographs in the American Pharmacopoeia has followed the proposal of the devices. In 1970, the American Pharmacopoeia presented drug release tests in only 12 monographs, all for the solid pharmaceutical form. This number changed to 462 in 1990, 630 in 2002 and approximately 787 in 2006, of which only 02 were for transdermal systems (clonidine and nicotine) (American Pharmacopoeia, 2009). Despite this, there is no consensus on which of the methods described would be suitable for *in vitro* release of transdermal forms.

The current Brazilian Pharmacopoeia has approximately 116 monographs with drug release tests, all for solid pharmaceutical forms (Brazilian Pharmacopoeia, 2005).

During the 1990s, various guidelines were drawn up by the FDA, FIP (*International Pharmaceutical Federation*) and EMEA (*European Medicines Agency*) covering most aspects of drug release trials (MANADAS *et al.,* 2002).

The scientific literature describes *in vitro* methods that mimic the process of transdermal release and penetration *in vivo* (AKAZAWA *et al.,* 1989) with and without membranes (artificial or biological) and different types of diffusion cells (AIACHE, 1992) of which Franz's *Vertical Diffusion Cell* (VDC) in a static and continuous flow system has been the most widely used in pharmacotechnical development, biopharmaceutical characterization and quality control, both for transdermal patches and semi-solid pharmaceutical forms (SHAH *et al.* 1994).

The apparatus of the diffusion cell in a static system consists of six thermoheated glass cells, a vat with receiving medium for replenishing the medium during sampling, a propeller for stirring the receiving medium, an automatic collector and a support for occluding the diffusion cell, which minimizes the effects of sample evaporation (**Figure 3**).

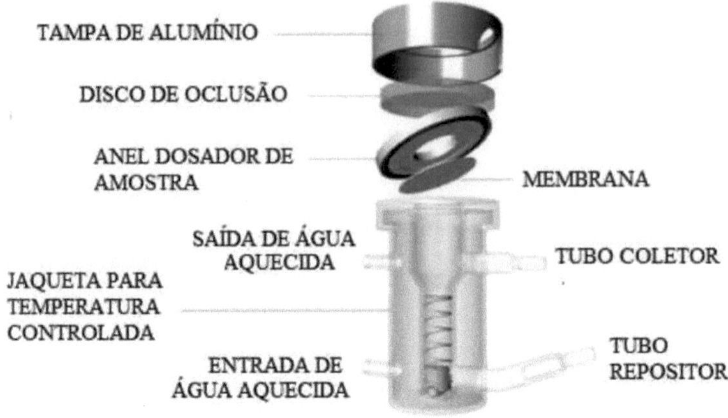

Figura 3. Image of the modified Franz VDC (*Hanson Corporation*).

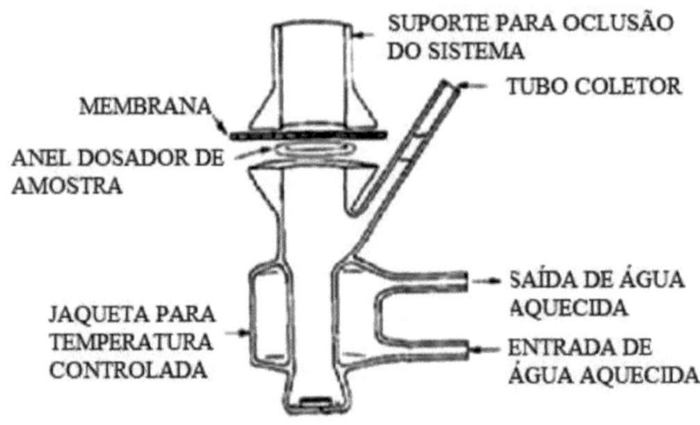

Figure 4 - Image of the VDC proposed by *Franz, 1975.*

Most articles using diffusion cells are based on Franz's publications in the mid-1970s (FRANZ, 1975, 1978). The Modified Franz cell was introduced in 1975 by FRANZ and is characterized by being a static, finite-dose diffusion cell, where the skin is mounted on a VDC and the dermis is in contact with a receptor sole (**Figure 4**). A quantity of the formulation to be studied is applied to the skin, mimicking *in vivo* conditions (BRONAUGH & STEWART, 1985). The volume of the receptor compartment is relatively large to ensure homogeneous soaking and dilution of the permeated substance (FRANZ, 1975).

The temperature of the system is controlled and maintained by a thermostated bath circulating through a jacket that surrounds the receiving chamber, the homogeneous distribution of temperature in the receiving room is achieved by the use of magnetic bars controlled by external magnetic stirrers (SARTORELLI *et al.,* 2000).

The Franz VDC in static system has been applied in various skin permeation studies, including transdermal and topical release formulations as well as cosmetics, pesticides and ophthalmics. According to *FDA Guideline SUPAC SS*, this system is ideal for quality control of topical preparations (FDA, 1997).

The Franz DCV with continuous flow is very similar in composition to the Franz DCV with static flow, but in this system the receiving solution is pumped continuously at a constant flow through an infusion pump (**Figure 5**).

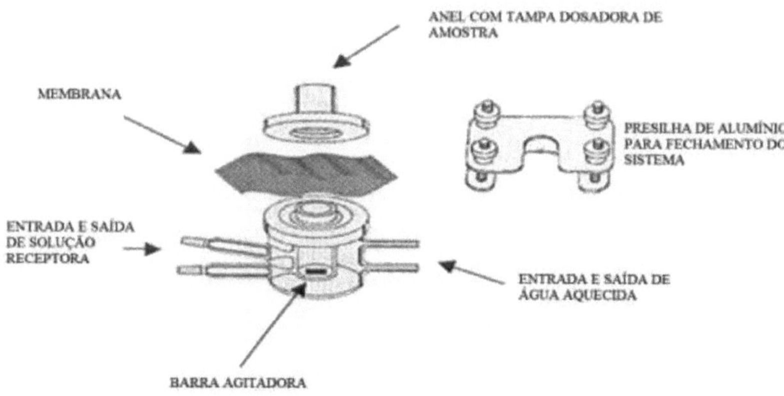

Figure 5: Schematic representation of the continuous flow diffusion cell.

Composition of the glass cell with a permeation area of 0.8 cm2 and a total volume of 3 mL.

Bronaugh and Steward (1985) introduced the continuous flow system to automate the cell sampling process by mimicking the blood flow of the skin, which is as close to the real thing as possible when compared to static systems. It was therefore able to monitor the drug release profile by sampling over a 24-hour period, as well as the maintenance of the *sink condition* throughout the experiment period (SARTORELLI *et al.*, 2000).

In September 2009, a forum of the American Pharmacopoeia suggested the use of VDC for quality control testing of topical and transdermal products (Pharmacopeial Forum, 2009).

To date, there is no method set out in official compendia for carrying out drug release tests on transdermal patches using Modified Franz VDC. However, the *FDA's Guidance for Industry on Scale up and Post Approval Changes for Semisolid* (SUPAC-SS) *dosage forms*, describes the study of *in vitro* release rate using Franz VDC for semi-solids and the American Pharmacopoeia published a Forum in 2009 indicating the use of VDC for hydrocortisone in semi-solid pharmaceutical form with analytical determination by HPLC (Pharmacopeial Forum, 2009).

The use of Franz CDV has also been widely described in the literature, in the development of new drug release systems (GARCIA *et al.,* 2004; ELVIRA *et al.,* 2003), new skin absorption promoters (LOPES *et al.,* 2005; JIA-YOU, 2003) and even suggesting new methods for official compendia.

Due to the great variability of formulations and their influence on drug release, as well as the diversity of application sites, a single official method would not be feasible for the development, biopharmaceutical characterization and quality control of all commercially available semi-solid and transdermal pharmaceutical forms. However, Franz's VDC can be considered the most promising apparatus for investigating changes after drug registration (FARE & ZATZ, 1995).

1.4.2. Parameters related to methodologies for in vitro release tests of topical and transdermal preparations

The *in vitro* transdermal release rate of a drug can be strongly influenced by parameters added to the methodology being applied in the release assay (SHAH & ELKINS 1995), thus explaining the large number of studies to validate the most effective and safe *in vitro* methodology mimicking the *in vivo* effects of drug release (ANSEL *et al.,* 2000). In this respect, Shah (1999) described the influence of parameters relating to the methodology, such as the composition of the receptor medium, the speed of agitation of the receptor medium and the batch difference of the synthetic membrane used *in in vitro* release tests for topical formulations. The methodology and apparatus to be used should contain characteristics that best describe the drug release and the release systems to be tested (SHAH, 1999).

The selection of an appropriate receptor medium is a critical factor in the success of the drug release experiment (SHAH *et al.,* 1994). The composition of the receptor medium must be able to maintain the *sink condition* at a temperature of 32 °C (± 0.5), be presented as a buffer solution with physiological pH for water-soluble drugs or as a hydro-alcoholic medium for lipophilic drugs. The use of surfactants in the receiving medium is acceptable as long as it is justified (FDA, 1997). When the concentration of the drug dissolved in the release medium is less than 10% of its saturation concentration, the system is said to be operating under *sink condition* (SINKO, 2008). The samples collected must have at least 5 different collection times throughout the period to determine the release flow (SHAH *et. al.,* 1999).

1.4.3. Membranes for in vitro release and skin permeation studies of topical and transdermal preparations

Human skin from plastic surgery would be ideal models for *in vitro* drug penetration studies through the skin. However, the limited availability of this type of material, the need to submit the experiment to the Ethics Committee and the difficulties and costs of storage, as well as the viability of this membrane model make its use limited (RIGG & BARRY, 1990; BABY *et al.*, 2008). As alternative membranes for human skin, researchers use experimental animal skin, synthetic membranes and three-dimensional cultures, such as reconstructed epidermis, called equivalent skin (ALIBERTI et al., 2017; PETRILLI et al., 2016; DEPIERI et al., 2015; ASCENO et al., 2015, 2014, 2013; CAMPOS et al., 2015; ESTRACANHOLLI et al., 2014; PETRILLI et al., 2013; TIOSSI et al., 2014; PRAÇA et al., 2012, 2011).

Pig ear skin has been recommended for *in vitro* skin permeation studies, because it has physiological, histological, hair follicle density and biochemical similarities to human skin (HAIGH and SMITH, 1994).

Some comparative studies of skin permeation in human skin, pig ear skin and other tissues including hairless mice are found in the literature, in which the results indicate pig ear skin as the most promising membrane model for *in vitro* permeation tests (FANG *et al.*, 1995).

Schomook, Meingassner and Billich (2001) compared the permeation properties of drugs with different polarities in human skin, pig ear skin, rat skin and reconstructed human epidermis (SkineethicTM). The authors concluded that pig ear skin seems to be the most suitable model, in the absence of human skin, where the flow and concentration of drugs through/in pig ear skin were of the same magnitude when compared to human skin.

Barbero and Frasch (2009) showed that both pigskin and Indian pigskin are good membrane models for replacing human skin and have lower variability values between them. They also concluded that the choice of the best membrane model will depend on the research proposal to be carried out.

In the last decade, there has been growing interest in the use of snakeskin seedlings as substitute models for human skin *in in vitro* drug permeation tests, and researchers have evaluated their applicability, obtaining favorable results (BABY *et al.*, 2007; ITOH *et al.*, 1990a; ITOH *et al.*, 1990b; RIGG and BARRY, 1990; WIDLER, SIGRIST and GAFNER, 2002). Snakeskin seedlings are composed of pure stratum corneum devoid of viable epidermis and hair follicles (RIGG, BARRY, 1990). It provides a barrier similar to the human stratum corneum and can be obtained in abundance without the death of the animal, since skin changes (or ecdysis) occur regularly in adult animals, usually every 2 to 3 months. The fact that it doesn't contain living tissues, it has no tendency to microbiological contamination and degradation, which makes it easy to store (ITOH *et al.*, 1990a,b; WIDLER, SIGRIST, GAFNER, 2002).

WIDLER, SIGRIST AND GAFNER (2002) demonstrated that snakeskin seedlings have similarities with the human stratum corneum, such as: tissue thickness (human CE - 13 to 15 μm; snake skin seedling - 10 to 20 μm); protein structure (keratin type α and β); lipid composition (human stratum corneum - 2.0 to 6.5%; snake skin seedling - approximately 6.0%, involving the presence of cholesterol, free fatty acids, glycoceramides and phospholipids, among others).

Snake skin has three distinct layers in its structure, including the outermost layer made up of beta-keratin, an intermediate layer also known as the meso layer, made up of intracellular alpha-keratin, which is considered to be similar to the human stratum corneum, and an intercellular lipid layer known as the inner layer. Itoh et al. (1990a) and Takahashi et al. (1993) identified the intermediate or *meso* layer as the main obstacle to the permeability of substances.

The snake skin molt is made up of two distinct regions, the dorsal region and the ventral region (**Figure 6**), in which the scales on the back are smaller than those on the ventral region (HAIG *et al.*, 1988). Itoh *et al.*, 1990a compared the permeation efficiency of *obsolete Elaphe* snake skin seedlings with human skin and observed that, considering the similarities between the skins tested, the ease of storage and handling, as well as the low cost of obtaining them, snake skin seedlings presented themselves as an alternative for replacing human skin *in in vitro* research into transdermal products.

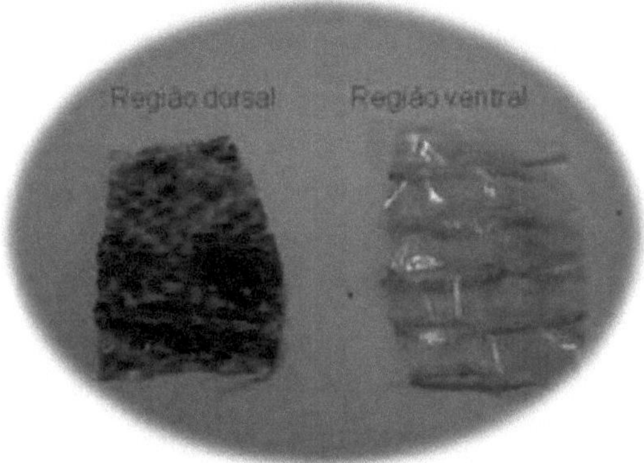

Figura 6. Image of the dorsal and ventral regions of the skin of *Crotalus durissu* snake seedlings, generously donated by the Central Bioterium of the USP Campus in Ribeirao Preto.

Pongjanyakul *et al.* (2002) observed that the evaporation flow of water from snake skins, when compared to human skin, is also very similar, although the permeability of water through the snake skin of various species is especially dependent on habitat conditions. In general, however, there is a great similarity in water permeability between snake skin molts and the human stratum corneum.

Baby *et al.* (2008) evaluated the physical, physico-chemical, chemical and functional stability of a cosmetic emulsion containing rutin and propylene glycol, as a skin penetration promoter, as well as the in vitro skin penetration and retention of this active ingredient, using *Crotalus durissu* snake skin seedlings as a biomembrane model. According to the results, the emulsion did not favor the skin penetration of rutin, but only its retention in the stratum corneum *of Crotalus durissus* skin.

Nunes *et al.* (2005) used *Boa constrictor* snake skins and human skin as a barrier for the *in vitro* permeation of transdermal indomethacin. The results showed a narrow variation in the coefficient of variation and in the reproducibility of the permeation profiles. The dorsal and ventral regions of snake skin have shown differences in diffusion characteristics (AIACHE *et al.*, 1998 and TAKAHASHI *et al.*, 2001).

1.5 *IN VITRO* SKIN PERMEATION

In vitro skin permeation tests have become one of the most important studies of topical and transdermal drug administration, with the aim of characterizing the permeation profile of formulations during pharmacotechnical development, as well as in batch-to-batch quality control (BARRY, 1983).

The *in vitro* procedure for the study of skin permeation generally involves the diffusion of the drug by concentration gradient through the membrane into a receiving solution where the analytical determination of the permeated drug content over time will be carried out (ALLEN *et al.*, 2008).

The diffusion of the drug through the skin can occur by three different routes: through the hair follicles associated with the sebaceous glands; through the ducts of the sweat glands and through the stratum corneum (**Figure 7**).

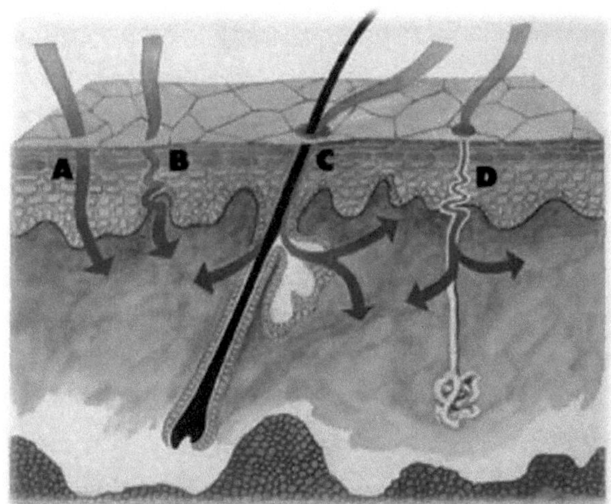

Figura 7. Schematic model of skin penetration pathways (A) intracellular stratum corneum, (B) intercellular stratum corneum, (C) hair follicle and (D) sebaceous duct (Thomas Spencer, 2009. www.aaps.com).

These different routes for the skin permeation of drugs have been debated for many years. The contribution of the skin appendage area to drug permeation is practically negligible since it accounts for 0.1% of the total skin permeation area, but this route is important for very polar molecules and for the specific administration of drugs in the hair follicle (BARRY, 2001).

Tregear (1961) discussed the influence of follicular transport on the cutaneous permeation of drugs. Elias *et al.* (1975) suggest that the intercellular route of the stratum corneum is a complex structure, rich in lipids, which may play an important role in percutaneous transport.

However, penetration through the stratum corneum occurs mainly via two routes: the intercellular route, where the drug diffuses around the corneocytes through the intercellular lipid matrix; and the transcellular route, where the drug passes through the corneocytes and the lipid matrix.

Since the route of permeation through intercellular channels is significant for the transport of drugs through the skin, it can be inferred that the stacking of corneocytes in the stratum corneum may dictate the length of the active's diffusion route through the skin. Thus, resistance to transport through the stratum corneum depends on the arrangement and properties of the alternating hydrophobic and hydrophilic layers of the stratum corneum, as well as its thickness, which varies from species to species and from body region to body region in the same individual. Several reports in the literature describe the influence of these factors on skin permeation. Rothman (1943) presented the scientific community with a review article in which he demonstrated that the carrier of the active ingredient, as well as the lipids in the skin, have a significant impact on the absorption and permeation rates of drugs. Hadgraft (2005), also in an article reviewing the scientific literature, demonstrated that skin permeability can vary from region to region. Smith *et al.* (1961) demonstrated greater permeability using skin from the scrotal region when compared to skin from the abdominal region for a series of drugs studied. The high permeability of this region has been used in transdermal systems containing testosterone. One of the most comprehensive studies of regional variation in skin permeability was carried out by Feldmann and Maibach (1967), who demonstrated the high permeability of the scrotal skin using cortisol as a model drug (FELDMANN and MAIBACH, 1967).

Other literature reviews on skin permeability were highlighted during the 1950s (HADGRAF & SOMERS, 1956; TREHEME, 1956). The advances in scientific research and understanding of the process of drug permeation through the skin during the 1950s and 1960s were due to efforts to understand the compositional properties of skin permeation barriers and how these properties can be systematically and reversibly modified.

1.5.1 Physico-chemical factors involved in skin permeation

The fundamental concepts that define the role of physicochemistry in the diffusion of drugs through the skin and mathematical models for evaluating the process of skin permeation remained in evidence during the 1960s with influential works published by Higuchi (1960).

A physical-chemical principle demonstrated by Higuchi (1960) highlights the influence of thermodynamic activity on the skin permeation of drugs. Coldman *et al.* (1969), following these concepts, developed topical formulations with volatile solvents. As the solvent evaporated, the vehicle became supersaturated and promoted greater thermodynamic transient activity (or chemical potential). This was the precursor to much of the work carried out in the 1990s.

The increasing progress in understanding the process of transdermal permeation is the result of research into the application of sensitive and sophisticated biophysical techniques. However, it is clear that some of these techniques have been applied for more than 40 years. For example, the infrared technique (ATR) was used to verify the action of components of the formulation vehicle on the skin surface (FISCHMEISTER *et al.*, 1975).

In the early 1970s, studies to measure skin conductivity by impedance measurements were described (WOOLLEY-HART, 1972) and at the end of the same decade, the application of nuclear magnetic resonance (NMR) with a diffusion probe in the stratum corneum, promoting the identification of various forms of water, was reported (PACKER & SELLWOOD, 1978). At the same time, transmission electron microscopy (TEM) was used to investigate ultrastructural details of the skin (BENTLEY *et al.*, 1997). More recently, DEPIERI et al. (2015) described various bioanalytical techniques for assessing the structure of the skin as well as the presence of drugs in the different layers of the skin, including fluorescence microscopy, confocal microscopy, multi-photon microscopy, Raman microscopy and Fourier transform mass spectrometry, among others.

1.6 NICOTINE TRANSDERMAL SYSTEMS: nicotine as a model drug

Transdermal nicotine delivery systems have been widely used in clinical protocols and therapeutic guidelines to replace nicotine in cigarette addiction (FANT *et al.,* 1999, SAUL *et al.,* 2007). Nicotine has several characteristics that make it an ideal drug for transdermal delivery systems. It is a diprotic base with pKa1 = 3.12 (pyridine ring) and pka2 = 8.02 (pyrrolidine ring), the structure of which is shown in **Figure 8.** It is highly soluble in polar and apolar solvents and has a low molecular mass, which theoretically makes it an efficient penetrant (SARA *et al.*, 1999).

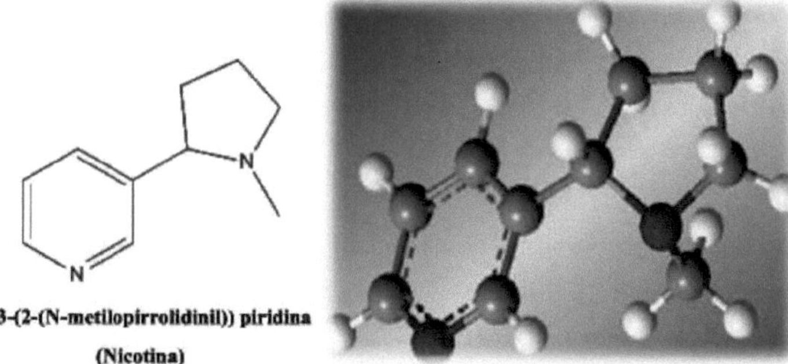

Figure 8. Molecular structure of nicotine (www.quimicaorganica.net)

In 1809, Vauquelin, a French scientist, was the first person to identify the molecule nicotine. He noticed the volatility and alkaloid activity in tobacco stratum. It wasn't until 1828 that it was isolated and purified by Poselt and Reimann at the University of Heildelberg. They named nicotine after Jean Nicot, one of the first people to import tobacco into France from "West India" in 1560 (FANT *et al.,* 1999).

In 1843 and 1847, Melsens established the empirical molecular formula for nicotine: $C_{10}H_{14}N_2$, and

Schloesing established its molecular mass: 162.23 g.mol^{-1}. It was only in 1895 that Adolf Pinner proposed the structure of nicotine known today (ROSEMBERG, 2003) (**Figure 8**).

The absorption of nicotine through cell membranes depends on pH. Assuming that nicotine's pKa2 is around 8.5, at acidic pH nicotine is ionized and does not easily cross membranes. However, at physiological pH (pH~7.4), 31% of nicotine is found in the non-ionized form, easily crossing membranes (GORROD, 1995).

In its basic form, nicotine is strongly alkaline and easily soluble in both water and lipids. In its ionized form, nicotine is more difficult to absorb. For this reason, alkaline media, in which nicotine is less ionizable, increase its bioavailability. In smokers, nicotine is administered orally. In people who do not inhale tobacco smoke, the main route of nicotine administration is through the nasal mucosa. However, absorption via this route is highly pH-dependent (BENOWITZ 1986, SVERSSON 1987).

Smokers who inhale cigarette smoke achieve greater absorption of nicotine through the small airways and alveoli, regardless of pH, and the mechanism by which this happens has not yet been fully elucidated (SARA *et al.,* 1999).

Nicotine replacement therapy is considered a safe method of treating smoking addiction, and is the most popular and least expensive. When compared to placebo, it is more effective and also influences the frequency of relapses (BENOWITZ *et al.*, 1998, STAPLETON *et al.,* 1995 and HUGHES *et al.*, 1999). This treatment can be applied using four forms of nicotine product: chewing gum, transdermal system, nasal spray and oral vaporizer (RIGOTTI *et al.,* 1999).

Chewing gum and the transdermal nicotine patch are available in Brazil. The counseling that accompanies nicotine replacement therapy is not intensive and, when administered to healthy adults, has produced positive results (JORENBY *et al.,* 1996; SHIFFMAN *et al.,* 1997). The use of this therapy alleviates the symptoms of withdrawal syndrome (RIGOTTI *et al.,* 1999; ROUSSEL *et al.,* 1997). With this treatment, remission can last six months or more (FOULDS *et al.,* 1993).

When nicotine replacement therapy is combined with other therapeutic resources (counseling or other medication), the effectiveness of the treatment can increase (RIGOTTI *et al.,* 1999).

At the moment, one of the drugs considered to be first-line in the treatment of nicotine dependence used in Brazil is the TTS patches containing nicotine (Ministry of Health, 2001). Patches of 7 mg, 14 mg and 21 mg of active nicotine are commercially available and can be used for an average of eight weeks. This form of nicotine replacement is the most suitable, as it has fewer side effects.

The dose reduction is progressive for up to a year. The patches must be changed every 24 hours and do not prevent the individual from playing sport. The most common side effect is skin irritation, which can prevent treatment from continuing. In Brazil, NiQuitin™ is the only transdermal patch for tobacco substitution therapy on the market.

These patches are available in three dosages: 21 mg, containing 114 mg of nicotine and releasing

21 mg/day; 14 mg, containing 78 mg of nicotine and releasing 14 mg/day; and 7 mg, containing 36 mg of nicotine and releasing 7 mg/day of nicotine. Each dosage is available in packs of 7 or 14 patches (sets for one or two weeks), in individual cartons.

Each NiQuitinTM adhesive has different layers made up of ethylene vinyl acetate copolymer, polyethylene terephthalate/vinylethylene acetate, polyisobutylene, polyethylene film, siliconized polyester film and printing ink (www.niquitin.com.br).

The patch should be applied to the skin, rotating the application site every 24 hours. For women, it should be avoided on the breast, and for men, it should be avoided on areas with hair. The area should be protected from direct sunlight, but there are no restrictions on use in water (BU0201/02).

The most common side effects in the groups treated with NiQuitin™ were generally abnormal dreams, arthralgia, colds, dry mouth, increased cough, insomnia, myalgia, nausea and pharyngitis. Those that may be related to nicotine are: abnormal dreams, dry mouth, dyspepsia, insomnia and nausea. Those that may be related to stopping smoking include arthralgia, colds, cold syndrome, myalgia and pharyngitis (BU0201/02).

In view of the bibliographical review, research into *in vitro* release methods and comparative analyses between them becomes valid, with the aim of stipulating specific criteria for the best choice *in the* use of methods and apparatus for *in vitro* studies of topical and transdermal drug release and permeation. Transdermal nicotine release systems can be considered models for this research.

2. OBJECTIVES

2.1 GENERAL OBJECTIVE

The aim of this project was to carry out and correlate *in vitro* nicotine release and permeation tests on commercially available transdermal patches, using the method indicated by the FDA (pads on disk) and the static and continuous flow Franz VDC, as well as validating the *in vitro* skin permeation and retention techniques with comparative intra- and inter-laboratory studies using biological membranes.

2.2 SPECIFIC OBJECTIVES

2.2.1 Development and validation of an analytical methodology for nicotine quantification using high performance liquid chromatography - HPLC.

2.2.2 Evaluation of the impact factors on the variability of *in vitro* release tests using the powder on disk method (FDA) and Franz VDC.

2.2.3 Evaluation of *in vitro* release using different methods: powder on disk (FDA), Franz VDC in a static system and continuous flow.

2.2.4 Evaluation of the *in vitro* permeation profile of nicotine using different membranes and methods.

2.2.5 Evaluation of the edge effect on *in vitro* release and permeation using Franz VDC in static and continuous flow systems.

2.2.6 Evaluation of *in vitro* retention in the skin layers (EC and [EP +D]) using the FDA and VDC method in a static system with different nicotine extraction techniques.

2.2.7 Analysis of the results obtained using different mathematical and statistical models.

3. MATERIAL AND METHODS

3.1 MATERIAL

- High Efficiency Liquid Chromatograph - Shimadzu SCL-10 A, LC Pump - 10 AD, Uv-Vis Detector SPD - 10 AD, Automatic Injector SIL - 10 AD.
- Chromatographic column - Lichrospher RP18-Select B, lot 186018.
- Vankel Dissolutor, model 7010, Dissolutor SR8 PLUS; Vankel apparatus for transdermal release - transdermal patch holder 2.5 part no. 12-4300.
- Franz VDC with static flow - Hanson Corporation.
- VDC with continuous flow and Spectra/Chromo CF-1 Fraction Collector.
- NiQuitinTM 78 mg, batch 071378814 and batch 062635714.
- Nicotine standard 1-methyl-2-3-pyridylpyrrolidine, batch 29H0467, SIGMA.
- Caffeine anhydrous standard batch 42207214 - Sigma Chemical Co.
- Leica cryostat microtome, model 1900.

3.2 METHODS

3.2.1 . Validation of the analytical methodology for nicotine quantification by High Performance Liquid Chromatography - HPLC

The methodology used was based on the conditions specified by PEREIRA *et al.* (2001) and validated in accordance with Resolution 310 of the National Health Surveillance Agency (2004), evaluating the parameters of linearity, intra and inter-test precision and accuracy, limit of quantification, limit of detection and robustness.

Specificity and Selectivity

Samples that could interfere with nicotine analysis were analyzed, such as the drug dilution solution (methanol), mobile phase (methanol: acetonitrile: acetic acid: acetate cap pH 4.5; 38:38:2:20 v/v), phosphate cap solution

(PBS) pH 7.4 (± 0.2) which was used as the receptor medium, methanolic solution containing EC on adhesive tapes and methanolic solution containing EP+D.

Each interfering sample was tested using the procedure and chromatographic conditions proposed in the analytical method for nicotine. The results were compared with those obtained with methanolic nicotine solution to check for peaks at the same retention time.

Chromatographic conditions

The equipment used was a high efficiency liquid chromatograph, operating with the aid of a column chromatogràfica select B - RP 18, Ultra-violet detector at 254 nm at a temperature of 35° C. The mobile phase used was composed of methanol: acetonitrile: acetic acid: acetate buffer pH 4.5 (38:38:2:20 v/v), adjusting the pH to 5.0 with diethylamine. The phase flow rate was around 1.0 mL/min and the injection volume was 50 μL. The samples were quantified using the nicotine peak areas.

Linearity and calibration curve

A calibration curve was prepared for nicotine containing six different concentrations, including the lower limit of quantification (LLQ).

The calibration curve was obtained from the nicotine stock solution, which was prepared by weighing 0.05 mg of the standard (1-methyl-2-3-pyridylpyrrolidine) and solubilizing it in a 10 mL volumetric flask with methanol. This solution had a final concentration of 5000 μg/ml of methanol.

From this solution, successive dilutions were made in PBS phosphate buffer solution pH 7.4 (±0.2), to final concentrations of 1000, 500, 100, 10, 1, 0.5 and 0.1 μg/mL. The solutions were analyzed in duplicates and the results were analyzed using the least squares linear regression statistical method and the linear regression coefficient.

Precision and Accuracy

The repeatability of the method was checked using three different concentrations of the analytical curve, with a high concentration of 100 μg/mL, a medium concentration of 10 μg/mL and a low concentration of 0.5 μg/mL of nicotine, making three determinations per concentration.

Precision and accuracy were determined in the same run, called intra-assay precision and intra-assay accuracy, and in 3 different runs, called inter-assay precision and inter-assay accuracy (BRASIL, Agència Nacional de Vigilância Sanitària, 2004).

The accuracy results were expressed as the coefficient of variation (CV%) according to the formula below:

CV% = (standard deviation/average concentration determined) X 100

While the accuracy results were expressed as the ratio between the average concentration determined experimentally and the corresponding theoretical concentration, following the formula:

Accuracy = (average experimental concentration/theoretical concentration) X 100

Lower limit of detection (LID) and lower limit of quantification (LIQ)

The LID was established by analyzing known and decreasing nicotine solutions up to the lowest detectable level being 2 to 3 times higher than the baseline noise, while the LIQ was established by analyzing standard nicotine solutions containing decreasing concentrations up to the lowest quantified level with precision and accuracy.

Robustness

The robustness of the analytical methodology was evaluated by comparing the nicotine peak areas in a methanolic solution of 10 µg/mL injected before and after varying the temperature of the chromatographic column oven by± 1°C, varying the composition of the mobile phase and varying the batch of the chromatographic column. The tests were carried out in triplicate.

3.2.2 *In vitro* release tests

3.2.2.1 Validation of Franz VDC with continuous flow

Some critical parameters of the Franz VDC system with continuous flow, which are: the volume of receiving solution in the compartments, the flow to be pumped to the receiving compartment, the variability of the sampled volume and the degree of evaporation of the collected solution, were validated for the performance of *in vitro* release and permeation.

Validation of the volume of receiving solution in the diffusion cell chambers

The volume of the VDC cell chamber was determined gravitationally by filling it with distilled water. The density of water was assumed to be 1.0 g/mL.

Validation of the flow of receiving solution pumped into the compartment

To check the amount of receptor medium collected every 5 minutes and thus calculate the flow rate (mL/h), the peristaltic pump was set to different flow rates, which were 0.5, 1, 2, 5 and 8 rpm. A graphical representation of the pump speed with the flow rate (mL/h) was made, as well as the linear regression of the curves obtained. The reproducibility of the system was evaluated over 3 consecutive days.

Validation of the degree of evaporation of the collected solution

Exactly 3 mL of the receiving medium was used to check the degree of evaporation of the collected solution. After adding the receiving medium, the same tubes were weighed again to determine the exact volume added. The tubes were kept in the automatic collector for a total of 24 hours and then weighed again. The difference in weight between the weighings was taken as the amount of solution evaporated.

Assessing the variability of the volume sampled

Collection tubes were previously weighed and placed in the automatic collector. The experiment was conducted at 32°C, using distilled water as the receiving solution and a pump set at a rate of 3.0 mL/h. The automatic sampler was programmed to sample every 15 minutes for a period of 1 hour. After the collections were completed, the tubes were weighed again and the volume of solution collected was taken as the difference in the weights of the tubes before and after collection.

Temperature control of diffusion cells

The temperature in the diffusion cells was measured in the donor and recipient compartments after a period of 1 hour, using a thermometer. The experiment was conducted at 32°C and the solvent used was distilled water.

Evaluation of the permeation area.

The permeation areas in cm^2 of the continuous flow DCV were evaluated individually using the mathematical model of the circumference areas, according to Equation (2):

(Eq. 2)

$$A = \pi.R^2$$

Where A is the area in cm^2 to be identified, π= 3.1416 and R is the radius of the circle.

To identify the radius of the permeation circle, we used a ruler in centimeters and the value of the circumference's diameter, divided in half.

3.2.2.2 Validation of Franz's VDC in a static system

To carry out the *in vitro* release and permeation tests using static Franz VDC, the following parameters were validated: the volume of receptor solution in each of the 6 cells and the variability in the volume sampled by the automatic collector.

- **Evaluation of the volume of receiving solution in each cell**

The volume of the inside of the cells was determined gravitationally by filling them with distilled water. The density of water is assumed to be 1.0 g/mL.

Evaluation of the variability in the volume sampled by the automatic collector.

1.5 mL vials were previously weighed and placed in the automatic collector. The experiment was conducted at 32°C, using distilled water as the receiving solution and the automatic collector was programmed to sample every 15 minutes for 1 hour. After collection, the tubes were weighed again and the volume of water collected was taken as the difference in the weights of the tubes before and after collection.

- **Validation of the degree of evaporation of the collected solution**

Exactly 1 mL of the receiving medium was used to check the degree of evaporation of the collected solution. After adding the capping solution using a volumetric pipette, the same tubes were weighed again to determine the exact volume added. The tubes were kept in the automatic collector for a total of 24 hours and then weighed again. The difference in weight between weighings was taken as the amount of solution evaporated.

Temperature control of diffusion cells

The temperature in the diffusion cells was measured in the donor and recipient compartments after a period of 1 hour using a thermometer. The experiment was conducted at 32°C and the solvent used was distilled water.

Evaluation of the permeation area

The permeation areas in cm^2 of the Vankel metal apparatus for transdermal release were evaluated individually, according to the procedure and Equation (2) described above.

3.2.2.3 Validation of the powder on disk system using transdermal apparatus - Vankel

In order to guarantee the reproducibility of the tests carried out on the disk-on-disk system (FDA), both *in the* release and *in vitro* permeation studies, the volume of receptor solution in each of the 6 dissolver tanks was evaluated, as well as the permeation area of the metal apparatus for transdermal systems.

Evaluation of the volume of receiving water in the dissolver vats

The volume of the dissolver tank was determined by filling it with distilled water using a beaker. The density of the water was assumed to be 1.0 g/mL.

Temperature control in the dissolver cells

The temperature in the vats of the Hanson dissolver was measured after a period of 1 hour using a thermometer. The experiment was conducted at 32°C and distilled water was used as the receiving solution.

Evaluation of the permeation area

The permeation areas in cm2 of the Vankel metal apparatus (**Figure 9**) for transdermal release were evaluated individually, according to the procedure and Equation (2) described above.

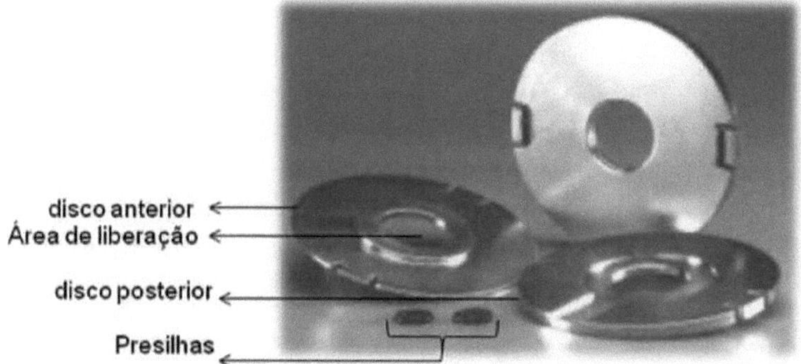

Figure 9. Illustrative image of the metallic release system for the Vankel transdermal patch (patent 5,108 710) part number 12-4300 with a release area of 2.5 cm2 (Vankel Technology Group, www.vankel.com).

1.1.1.4 Evaluation of the impact factors on the variability of the *in vitro* release assay using the FDA's foot-on-disc method and Franz's VDC

The tests were carried out in Dissolution equipment (**Figure 10**) with a Vankel apparatus (**Figure 9**) for the FDA method, as well as in static Franz VDC equipment, both at 32°C (± 0.5) and transdermal patches containing 78 mg of nicotine, commercially available in the NiQuitinTM 14 mg version.

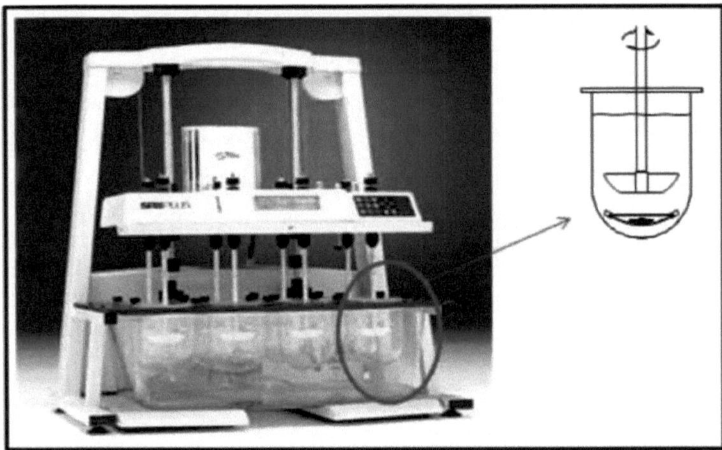

Figure 10. Illustrative image of the Hanson dissolution system and apparatus 5 (FDA) described by the American Pharmacopoeia (modified from www.flowscience.com.br and USP 29, 2006).

The transdermal patches were duly fitted to the discs of the Vankel metal system (FDA) and the Franz VDC, leaving only the determined area of 2.5cm and 1.77cm exposed to the receiving medium[2] respectively. Variability tests were then carried out.

The first test evaluated the influence of different receptor media on the *in vitro* release profile of nicotine in transdermal patches by stirring at 50 rpm with 900 mL of receptor volume in the powder on disk method (FDA). With this test, it was possible to reproduce the nicotine release methodology as suggested by the American Pharmacopoeia (USP) which indicates the use of aqueous media as well as acidic media in 0.025N HCL and compare with the release results in alkaline media, PBS buffer, pH 7.4 (±0.2).

The second test evaluated the influence of different batches of the drug (batch A and batch B). PBS phosphate buffer solution pH 7.4 (± 0.2) at 32°C (± 0.5), stirring at 50 rpm and a receiver volume of 900 mL were used for the dissolver and, for Franz VDC in a static system, stirring at 300 rpm and 7mL of receiver solution. The membrane used was pig ear skin dermatomized to a thickness of 500 µm.

The third test evaluated the influence of stirring speed on the dissolution medium. Isotonic phosphate buffer medium was used, PBS pH 7.4 (± 0.2) at 32°C (± 0.5), at different stirring speeds: 50, 75 and

100 rpm for the powder on disk method (FDA).

All the tests were carried out by collecting 1 mL of sample at pre-determined times of 1, 2, 3, 4, 6 and 8 hours and using n = 5, except for the agitation speed test which used n = 15 to favor statistical comparison calculations of f_1 and f_2. Exactly 50 µL were injected into the HPLC to quantify the nicotine released.

1.1.1.5 Evaluation of *in vitro* release using different apparatuses: powder on disk (FDA), Franz VDC in static and continuous flow system

After selecting the experimental conditions through the tests described above, the *in vitro* release tests were carried out using the powder on disk method (FDA), Franz VDC in a static and continuous flow system.

The receptor medium selected in section 3.2.2.4 was isotonic phosphate buffer pH 7.4 (±0.2) 0.01M, in different volumes according to the equipment model, 900 mL for powder on disk (FDA), 7 mL for VDC in a static system and 3 mL for VDC with continuous flow. The tests were carried out in the absence of a membrane and with n = 15.

3.2.3 *In vitro* permeation

3.2.3.1 Obtaining and dermatomizing pig ear skins.

The pig ears were obtained from the FRIPON slaughterhouse in the city of Pontal - SP and immediately sanitized with distilled water. The skin was then dissected from the dorsal region of the pig's ear and fixed to a horizontal support for dermatomization using a dermatometer.

The dermatomization process involved making a parallel cut in the skin surface, thus making the thickness of the tissue around 500 µm uniform. The dermatomized skins were frozen for a maximum of 30 days until they were used in the skin permeation tests.

3.2.3.2 Obtaining the hairless mouse skins

Hairless mice were obtained from the HRS/J strain, Jackson Laboratories, Bar Habor, ME -USA, females (22 to 28g), belonging to the Pharmaceutical Technology laboratory at FCFRP-USP.

The animals were euthanized by carbon dioxide vapor (according to protocol 09.1.505.53.6 - Ethics Committee on the Use of Animals), and after dissecting the skin, it was sanitized with distilled water. The skins were frozen for a maximum of 30 days until they were used in the skin permeation tests.

3.2.3.3 Obtaining snakeskin seedlings

Snake skin seedlings of the species *Crotalus durissus*, popularly known as the rattlesnake, from snakes aged approximately 2 years, were kindly donated by the Central Bioterium of the University of Sao Paulo - Ribeirao Preto Campus. After receiving the skin cuttings, they were immediately washed with an excess of distilled water, then the excess water was removed using a paper towel applied with gentle compression to the skin.

The drying process was completed at room temperature (25.0 ± 2.0 oc). The seedlings were stored and protected from light for less than 30 days before use, according to procedures described in the literature (BABY *et al.*, 2006b, BABY *et al.*, 2007b).

3.2.3.4 *In vitro* nicotine using different methods: bread on disk (FDA), static Franz VDC and with continuous flow

The skin permeation tests were carried out according to the method described by OECD 428 and the SCCP *Guideline*, both for Franz VDC in a static system (**Figure 4**) and continuous flow (**Figure 5**), as well as the foot-on-disc method (**Figures 9** and **10**).

The receptor medium used was isotonic phosphate buffer PBS pH 7.4 (± 0.2) 0.01M and the permeation membrane was pig ear skin dermatomized to approximately 500 μm.

The Franz VDC, in both static and continuous flow systems, was set up with the dermal region of the skin in contact with the receptor medium. The transdermal nicotine patch was placed in contact with the stratum corneum and kept under occlusion throughout the test.

The foot-on-disc method suggested by the FDA was mounted on a Hanson SR8 Plus Dissolver with a dissolving vat containing 900 mL of the same receptor medium (**Figure 10**). The skin was mounted between the metal Vankel disks (**Figure 9**) with the transdermal nicotine patch in contact with the EC while the receptor solution was in contact with the dermis.

For the tests carried out in VDC in a static system and the foot-on-disc method (FDA), 1mL of the receiving medium was collected at predetermined times of 2, 4, 6 and 8 hours, with the same volume of receiving medium being replaced. For the tests carried out in VDC in continuous flow, the flow speed was 0.5 rpm and the consequent flow rate was 3 mL/h.

After collecting the receptor solution, exactly 50 μL were injected into the liquid chromatograph to quantify the nicotine present, as described in section 3.2.1.

3.2.3.5 Evaluation of the influence of different membranes on the *in vitro* rate of nicotine using Franz VDC in a static system

The influence of different biological membranes on the *in vitro* rates of nicotine *in* a NiQuitinTM transdermal patch containing 78 mg of nicotine was evaluated, with the aim of verifying the dependence of the release system ά membrane on permeation.

The membranes tested were pig ear skin dermatomized to 500 μm, non-dermatomized hairless mouse skin and *Crotalus durissus* snake skin seedlings with 24 and 48 hours of hydration in distilled water.

The use of the ventral portions of *Crotalus durissus* skin seedlings was standardized as described by Baby *et al.* (2008), prior to carrying out the *in vitro* skin penetration study. Using the mechanical removal technique, the superficial layers of tissue were removed by applying adhesive tape only once (Scotch, 3M). They were then moisturized by immersion in distilled water at 25.0± 2.0 °C for

24 and 48 hours before use. After the skins were hydrated, they were cut into sizes suitable for the permeation tests and placed on the Franz VDC in a static system.

Dermatomized pig skin and hairless mouse skin were fixed in Franz VDC according to the procedure described in item 3.2.3.4. Permeation tests were carried out according to the method described in item 3.2.3.4 and the amount of nicotine permeated was quantified by CLAE according to item 3.2.1.

3.2.3.6 Evaluation of the edge effect on nicotine release and skin permeation *in vitro*

Additional *in vitro* release and permeation tests of the nicotine present in NiQuitin™ patches containing 78mg of nicotine were carried out with the transdermal patches untrimmed and trimmed to a diameter of 3.0 cm^2, which is suitable for promoting adhesion of the system to the Franz VDC. Release tests were conducted in the absence of a membrane, while permeation tests used pig ear skin dermatomized to approximately 500 μm. The test methodology was carried out as described in section 3.2.3.4 and the amount of nicotine permeated was quantified by HPLC in accordance with section 3.2.1.

3.2.3.7 Analytical quantification of *in vitro* permeation samples

The amount of nicotine present *in* the samples collected from the *in vitro* permeation test was determined by HPLC under the conditions described in section 3.2.1. Corrections for the dilution of the receptor phase were made using equation 3:

Eq(3)

$$Q_{real,\,t} = C_t \,.\, V_r + \quad \Sigma \quad V_c \,.\, C_c$$

where:

Q real, t = real quantity permeated at time t

Ct = concentration obtained at time t

Vr = volume of receiving solution

Cc = sampling concentration

Vc = volume sampled

The quantity permeated ($Q_{real,\,t}$) at a given t is equal to the quantity measured (Q_t), plus the quantities removed from the cell or vat during previous sampling and discarding.

3.2.4 *In vitro* skin retention

After 12 hours of *in vitro* permeation tests carried out according to item 3.2.3.4, the skins were removed from the Franz VDC using a static system and the foot-on-disc (FDA) method, with the transdermal adhesive gently removed. The pig ear skins were fixed on a smooth surface to remove the CE using the conventional *tape stripping* technique and then the amount of nicotine retained in the EP + D (without stratum corneum) was checked, according to the methodologies validated in section 3.2.3.4.

After extracting the nicotine retained in the skin, exactly 50 µL of the sample was analyzed by CLAE to quantify the nicotine present. The experiments were conducted with a total of 15 replicates.

3.2.4.1 Development and validation of the technique for extracting nicotine retained in pig ear skin through horizontal cuts at different depths of the total skin

The methodology for mapping nicotine retained in different depths of pig ear skin after 12 hours of permeation with NiQuitin™ transdermal patches containing 78mg of nicotine was developed at the end of the *in vitro* permeation experiments (item 3.2.3.5). The pig ear skins were removed from the static Franz VDC and the transdermal patch gently removed.

The skins were fixed to a smooth surface to select the permeation area (1.77cm^2) using a metal cutter in a cylindrical shape. The permeation areas were then frozen using O.C.T™ compound (Tissue - Tek®) and a cooled acetone bath. After freezing, the skins were then transferred to the cryostat microtome equipment, where horizontal cuts were made in the skin. Ten horizontal cuts were made, each with a thickness of 40 µm. Each cut was transferred to a test tube containing 1 mL of receptor medium for nicotine extraction using an ultrasonic bath for 15 min and a vertical mixer for 1 min. Then 50 µL of the supernatant was injected into a HPLC to quantify the nicotine present. The experiment was conducted in triplicate.

3.2.5 Mathematical models and statistical tests

3.2.5.1 Mathematical model for comparing *in vitro* release profiles using the Difference Factor (f_1) and Similarity Factor (f_2)

In this comparison we evaluate the release profile curve as a whole using a simple Independent Model Method in which a difference factor (f_1) and a similarity factor (f_2) are used. The f1 factor calculates the percentage difference between the two profiles evaluated at each collection time and corresponds to a measure of the relative error between the profiles.

Eq(4):

$$f_{(1)} = \left\{\left[\frac{\sum_{i=l}^{n}(R_f - T_t)}{\sum_{i=l}^{n} R_f}\right]\right\} x\ 100$$

where: n= number of collection times; R_f = dissolved percentage value at time t, obtained with the reference apparatus. Tt = dissolved percentage value of the product in the test equipment at time t.

The f2 factor corresponds to a measure of similarity between the dissolved percentages of both profiles.

Eq(5):

$$f_{(2)} = 50\ x \log\{[1 + \left(\frac{1}{n}\right) x \sum_{i=l}^{n} (R_f - T_t)^2]^{0,5} x\ 100\}$$

The criteria for two dissolution profiles to be considered similar are based on the results of the factors f1 = 0 to 15 and f2 = 50 to 100.

3.2.5.2 Statistical Tests

The results obtained in the *in vitro* nicotine release and skin permeation tests were expressed in graphs relating the amount released or permeated per area of exposure (µg/cm^2) as a function of collection time. Following this model, it was possible to identify the release kinetics and flows of nicotine release and permeation. The fluxes were calculated using the slope of the linear portion of the curve (*steady state*) presented as the average of 15 replicates.

The demonstration of the results in the form of percentage of nicotine released per cm^2 collection time was also used to enable comparative calculations of the difference (f1) and similarity (f2) factors.

The results obtained in this project, in terms of release, permeation and intra- and inter-laboratory validation, were compared using the ONEWAY ANOVA non-parametric statistical model, with a significance level of 0.05 ($p < 0.05$).

4. RESULTS

4.1 . Development and validation of analytical methodology for nicotine quantification by CLAE.

The development and validation of the analytical methodology for nicotine by High Performance Liquid Chromatography was carried out by determining the parameters of linearity, specificity, selectivity, precision, accuracy, limit of detection, limit of quantification and robustness of the methodology. The elution chromatograms of nicotine and possible interferents are shown in **Figure 11**.

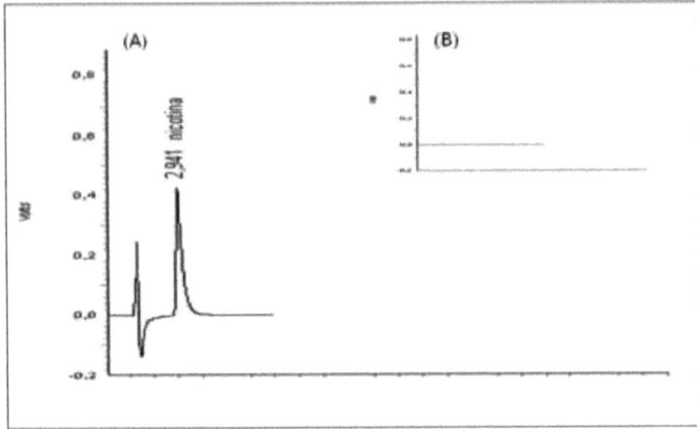

Figure 11. Chromatogram of the nicotine standard 100 µg/mL in methanol showing the drug's retention time (A) and chromatogram of possible interferents, such as: mobile phase, methanol and receptor medium (B), obtained using a reverse phase column (Select-B) RP18. The mobile phase used was composed of methanol: acetonitrile: acetic acid: acetate buffer pH 4.5 (38:38:2:20 v/v), adjusting the pH to 5.0 with diethylamine, a flow rate of 1.0 mL/min, an injection volume of 50 µL and ultraviolet detection at 254 nm.

The nicotine analytical curve is shown in **Figure 12** and was used for the validation analysis of the methodology as well as for the calculations of the release, permeation and skin retention samples.

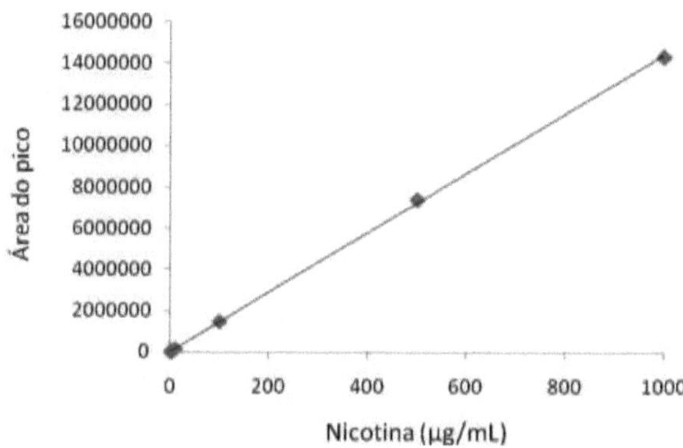

Figure 12. Representative graph of the nicotine analytical curve comprising concentrations from 0.1 to 1000 µg/mL by HPLC. The mobile phase used was methanol: acetonitrile: acetic acid: acetate buffer pH 4.5 (38:38:2:20 v/v) adjusting the pH to 5.0 with diethylamine and a Select B - Lichrospher RP 18 chromatographic column at 35°C and detection at λ= 254 nm.

Tables 1 and **2** show the linearity parameters, as well as the intra- and inter-test precision and accuracy of the analytical method. The linearity of the analytical curve showed a linear correlation coefficient of 0.999 with a coefficient of variation of 8.6%. The intra- and inter-assay precision and accuracy showed a maximum coefficient of variation of 3.4% and accuracy of over 95.8%.

Table 1. Linearity parameters of the analytical method for nicotine quantification by HPLC.

Parameters	Values obtained
Equation of the line	y = 7.08028e-005x+0
Linear correlation coefficient (r)	0,9999
Coefficient of determination (r^2)	0,9995
Quantification limit	0,1
Detection limit	0,05

The above values were obtained using the criteria specified in section 3.2.1.

Table 2. Precision and Accuracy values of the analytical methodology for nicotine quantification by HPLC.

(n = 3)	Low Concentration 0.5 µg/mL	Average concentration 10 µg/mL	High concentration 100 µg/mL
	Intra-test		
Average	0,48	9,58	98,82
Accuracy (%)	2,41	0,76	0,19

Accuracy (%)	97,80	95,89	98,82
Inter-assay			
Day 1	97,80	95,89	98,82
Day 2	100,3	96,84	99,22
Day 3	104,6	96,55	99,84
Average	100,9	96,55	99,29
Accuracy (Error) (%)	3,40	0,59	0,51
Accuracy (%)	100,9	96,55	99,29

The results of the robustness of the analytical methodology are shown in **Table 3.** The nicotine peak proved to be symmetrical and no coefficient of variation values greater than 7% were found in the peak area values for any of the proposed changes.

Table 3. Evaluation of the robustness of the analytical methodology for nicotine in HPLC by varying the composition of the mobile phase, the temperature and the batch of chromatographic columns.

Mobile phase methanol: acetonitrile: acetic acid: acetate cap pH 4.5			Chromatographic column Temperature		Lot	
	36:40:2:20	40:36:2:20	34°C	36°C	497117	165018
µg/mL	9,74 (± 0,01)	9,85(± 0,05)	9,98(±0,1)	10,41(±0,03)	9,85(±0,2)	9,81(±0,6)
CV (%)	0,102	0,507	1,001	0,288	2,029	6,113

(±) values representing the standard deviation of the analyses (n =3)

4.2 Evaluation of *in vitro* release

The validation results of the different methods used for the *in vitro* release and permeation tests are shown in **Table 4**. No coefficients of variation greater than 5% were observed. **Figure 13** shows the linear relationship between the volume collected and the speed of the infusion pump.

Table 4: Instrumental validation of the Franz VDC systems in both continuous flow and static systems and of the powder on disk method (FDA) used in the *in vitro* release and permeation tests.

	Continuous VDC	Static VDC	FDA paws on disk
Volume of receptor solution in cells and vats (mL)	3.8 (± 0.075) HP% = 1.96	7.3 (± 0.2) HP% = 2.7	900.1 (± 2.3) HP% = 0.25
Sample volume variability (mL)	3.51 (± 0.028) HP% = 0.81	1.0 (± 0.05) HP% = 5.0	1.0 (± 0.003) HP% = 3.0

Temperature control of cells and vats (°C)	32 (± 0.05) HP% = 0.15	32 (± 0.001) HP% =0.003	32.3 (± 0.01) HP% =0.03
Permeation area (cm2)	0.78 (± 0.005) HP% = 0.63	1.76 (± 0.02) HP% = 1.13	2.53 (± 0.08) HP% = 3.16
Degree of evaporation of the solution collected after 24 hours (%)	1.0 (± 0.02) CV% = 2.0	0.09 (± 0.001) HP% = 1.1	1.1 (± 0.01) CV% = 0.9

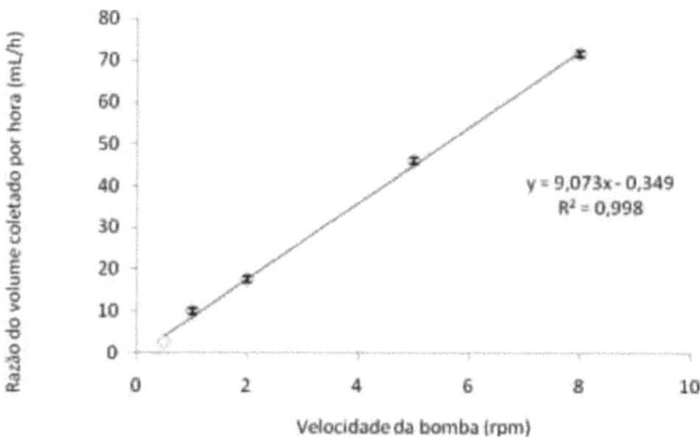

Figura 13. Representation of the linearity in the ratio of the pumping flow of receiver solution into the Franz VDC compartment with continuous flow, using different speeds (0.5, 1, 2, 5 and 8 rpm).

4.3 Evaluation of the impact factors on the variability of the *in vitro* release test using the powder on disk method (FDA) and VDC with static flow.

To assess the influence of the composition of the receptor medium on nicotine release, different media were tested, including 0.01M PBS pH 7.4 (± 0.2) phosphate buffer, deionized water and 0.025N HCl. The results are shown in **Figure 14**. The highest nicotine release values at 8 hours were obtained using the alkaline receptor medium PBS phosphate buffer pH 7.4 (± 0.2), 0.01M.

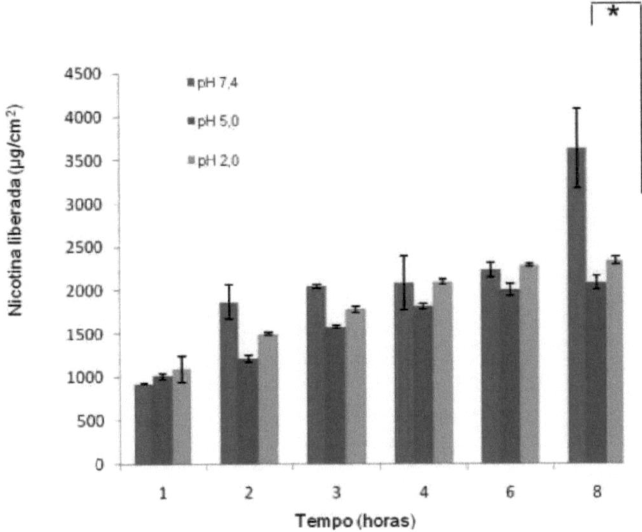

Figura 14. Nicotine release profile with accumulated amounts (μg/cm^2) as a function of time (hours), obtained in PBS phosphate buffer pH 7.4 (± 0.2) 0.01M, deionized water and HCl 0.025N, using a dissolver with a pad-on-disc apparatus (FDA method) and the presence of bars representing the standard deviation (n= 5). * Significant differences between PBS phosphate buffer and the other media tested ($p<0.05$).

Figure 15 shows the influence of the stirring speed of the receptor medium on the release of nicotine after 8 hours of testing. The cumulative amount of nicotine released in 8 hours showed no significant difference for the speeds of 50 and 75 rpm in the powder on disk method (FDA) and 300 rpm in VCD in a static system.

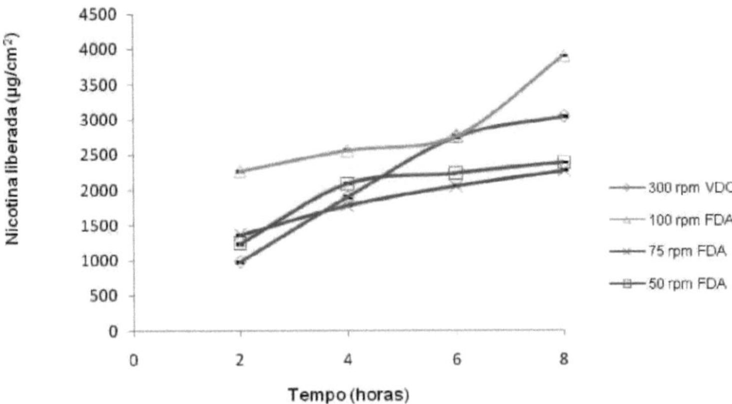

Figura 15. Nicotine release profile up to 8 hours of testing at different speeds of agitation of the

receptor medium (PBS phosphate buffer pH 7.4 (± 0.2) 0.01M), using Franz VDC (VDC), powder on disk method (FDA) and NiQuitinTM transdermal patches. The standard deviation bars are shown overlaying the signals (n = 15).

The results of the similarity in the release profile of the different batches of the drug NiQuitin™ containing 78mg of nicotine used in the permeation and skin retention tests were evaluated and are shown in **Figure 16.**

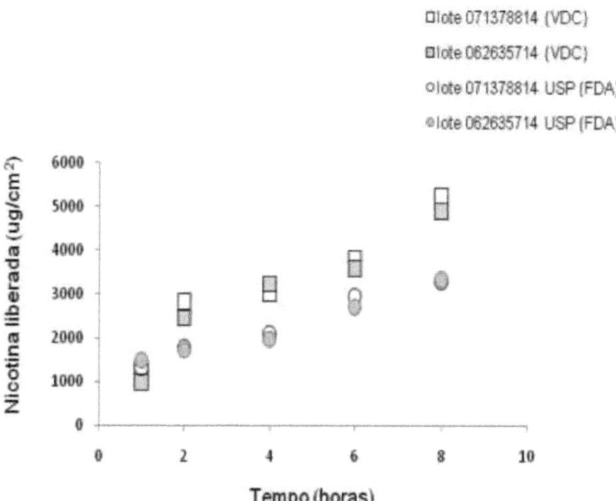

Figura 16. Nicotine release profile up to 8 hours of testing in receptor medium (PBS phosphate buffer pH 7.4 (± 0.2) 0.01M), using Franz VDC (VDC), powder on disk method (FDA) and different batches of NiQuitin™ transdermal patches. The standard deviation bars are shown overlaying the signals (n = 5).

The process of radial nicotine diffusion was evaluated in NiQuitinTM transdermal patch systems with a total area of 15 cm^2 and 5100 µg/cm^2 of nicotine. **Figures 17 A** and **B** show values of approximately 100 and greater than 100% of nicotine present in the experimental diffusion area (1.77 cm^2) over a release period of 8 and 12 hours respectively. In the permeation tests up to 8 hours, there was no significant difference between the trimmed and whole adhesives.

(A)

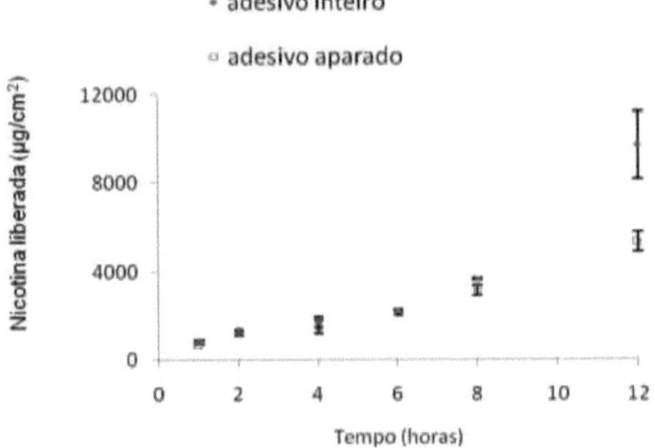

(B)

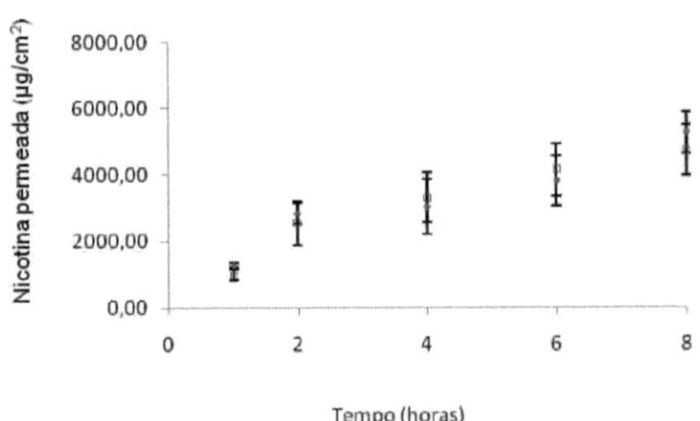

Figura 17. Release profile (A) and permeation (B) of nicotine present in NiQuitinTM transdermal patches containing 78 mg nicotine, whole (15 cm^2 area) and trimmed to 3.0 cm^2 using Franz VDC.

The results of the *in vitro* release of nicotine from transdermal patches were obtained using different methods, namely the FDA method, VDC in a static system and VDC with continuous flow, which are shown in **Figure 18**. All the methods tested showed results above 80% release up to 8 hours of release.

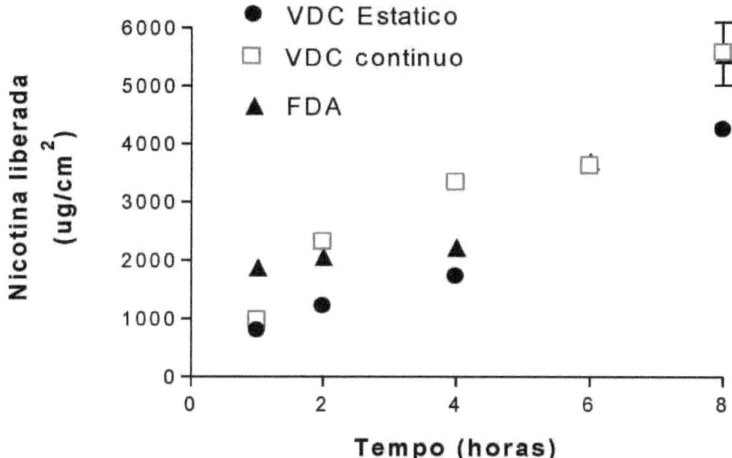

Figura 18. Nicotine release profile in the absence of a membrane. The tests were carried out in a foot-on-disc (FDA) method containing 900 mL of receptor phase at 50 rpm, static VDC containing 7 mL of receptor medium at 300 rpm, and VDC with continuous flow containing 3 mL of receptor phase at 300 rpm. The bars represent the standard deviation (n = 15).

Accumulated amounts of nicotine released in up to 8 hours were in the order of 5555.21 (±189), 4258.66 (±152) and 5572.0 (±138) µg/cm^2 for the foot-on-disc method (FDA), and VDC in static and continuous flow systems, respectively. While the flow values (*J*) calculated from the linear portion of the release curve were 510.5 (±49.8) for FDA, 494.3 (±15.3) for VDC in a static system and 574.8 (±23.2) for VDC with continuous flow.

The application of the mathematical model f_1 and f_2 to compare the release profiles of transdermal products is shown in **Table 5** and **Figure 19**.

However, these results showed similarities between the stirring speeds of 50 to 75 rpm for the powder on disk method (FDA) and 300 rpm for the Franz VDC in a static system; as well as between the release profiles with the VDC method in continuous flow and FDA.

Table 5. Demonstration of the factors of difference (f_1) and similarity (f_2) of the profiles obtained by the *in vitro* nicotine release tests at different speeds of agitation of the receiving medium in different equipment. *** Significant difference with $p>0.05$.

	Factor f_1	*Factor f_2*	*One-Way ANOVA (p>0.05)*
Agitatlon (rpm)			
50 FDA X 100 FDA	27,23	88,86	***
50 FDAX 75 FDA	9,75	98,50	$p < 0,05$

50 FDA X 300 VDC static	9,28	98,39	$p < 0,05$

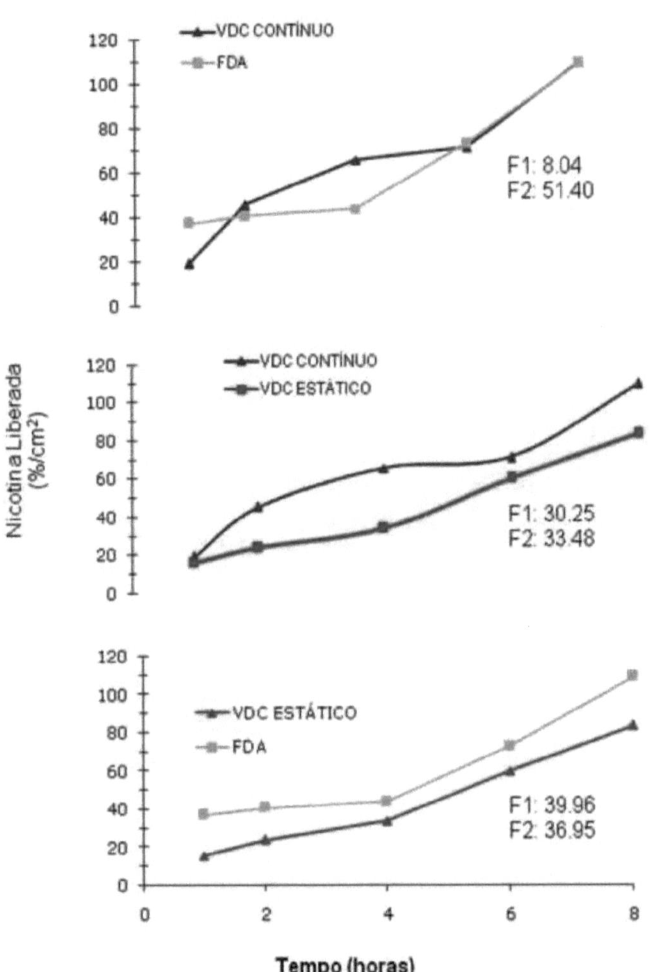

Figura 19. Graphical demonstration *in vitro* nicotine release profiles in %/cm^2 in a receptor medium, obtained using the FDA static VDC methods and with continuous flow for calculating the f_1 and f_2 factors.

4.4 Evaluation of *in vitro* permeation

The effect of the influence of different membranes on the *in vitro* permeation rate is shown in **Figure 20** and **Table 6**. It was possible to observe that the NiQuitinTM nicotine transdermal system has membrane-dependent permeation characteristics, since nicotine values in µg/cm^2 were found to be

2.3 times higher in 8 hours of permeation with biological membranes, when compared to the samples obtained in the absence of a membrane.

However, no significant difference was observed in the accumulated amount of nicotine permeated at 8 hours for pig ear skin, hairless mouse skin and snake skin moisturized for 24 hours.

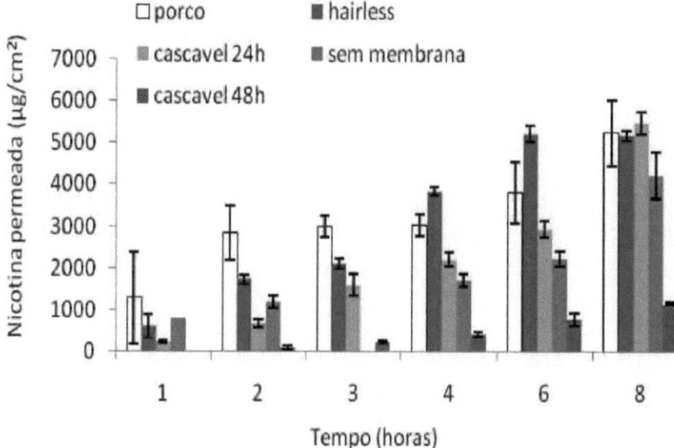

Figura 20. Nicotine permeation profile in the absence of a membrane and with different types of biological membranes (pig ear skin, hairless mouse skin and snake skin). The tests were carried out using the VDC method in a static system containing 7 mL of receptor medium at 300 rpm. The bars represent the standard deviation (n = 15).

The amounts of nicotine permeated in μg/cm^2 as well as the flow *(J= μg/cm^{2}h^{-1})* up to 8 hours of permeation were significantly lower for the feet on disk (FDA) method when compared to the results in VDC in both static and continuous flow systems (**Table 6**).

Table 6. Kinetic factors and comparison of permeation profiles using different equipment and biological membranes.

Membrane / Method	**Amount of nicotine permeated (μg/cm^2) in 8 hours**	**Permeation flux *J* = (μg/cm$^{(2)}$/h^{-1})**	**One-Way ANOVA (p>0.05) for (*J*)**
Without static membrane/VDC	4229.28 (±335) CV% = 7.90	250,7 (± 21,58)	***
Rattlesnake 24h hydration/VDC static	5488,7 (± 270) CV% = 4.9	710,7 (± 72,55)	p < 0,05
Rattlesnake 48h hydration/VDC static	1161,0 (± 31,55) CV% = 2.7	178,2 (± 4,68)	***

Hairless mouse skin / static VDC	5175,9 (± 121) CV% = 2.3	698,2 (± 116,7)	p < 0,05
Pigskin / static VDC	5246,0 (± 777,9) CV% = 14.8	813,1 (± 103,2)	p < 0,05
Pigskin /VDC continuous flow	4719,2 (± 333,02) CV% = 7.1	576,5 (± 110,4)	***
Pig ear skin /FDA	3294,1 (± 50,5) CV% = 1.5	339,7 (± 42,59)	***

(±) standard deviation of averages obtained from 5 experiments. The flux *(J)* was calculated from the slope *in* the linear portion (*steady state*) of the *in vitro* permeation curve after 8 hours.*** Significant difference with p>0.05.

Pig ear skin was selected as the model membrane for comparative evaluation of nicotine permeation *in vitro*. The results obtained using different methodologies such as the foot on disk method (FDA), static VDC and continuous flow VDC are shown in **Figure 21.**

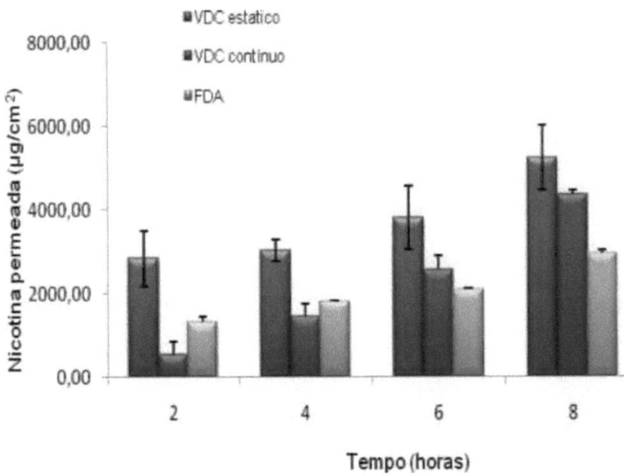

Figura 21. Nicotine permeation profile using pig ear skin. The tests were carried out in a foot-on-disc (FDA) method containing 900 mL of receptor phase at 50 rpm, VDC in a static system containing 7 mL of receptor medium at 300 rpm, and VDC with continuous flow containing 3 mL of receptor phase at 300 rpm. The bars represent the standard deviation (n = 15).

4.5 Evaluation of skin retention *in vitro*

The skin retention tests on the different layers of pig ear skin using VDC in a static system and the foot on disk method (FDA) are shown in **Figure 22**.

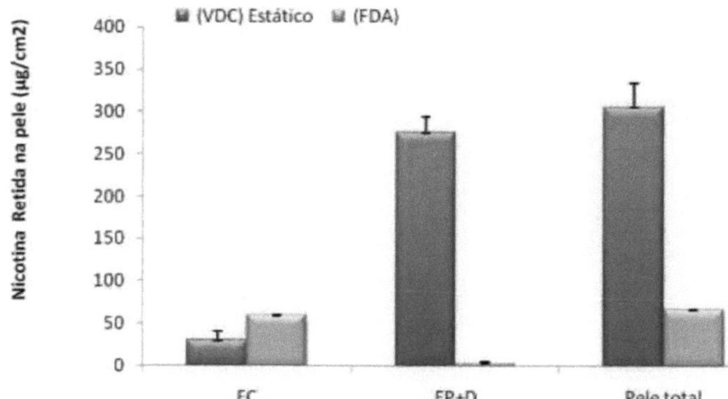

Figura 22. Amounts of nicotine retained in the different layers of pig ear skin (EC and EP+D) using methods, FDA and VDC in a static system, after 12 hours of permeation, with bars representing the standard deviation (n = 5).

The mapping of nicotine retention at different skin depths after 12 hours of skin permeation using VDC is shown in **Figure 23** and suggests that similar amounts of nicotine are present at every 40 µm of skin, indicating nicotine partitioning in all layers of the skin.

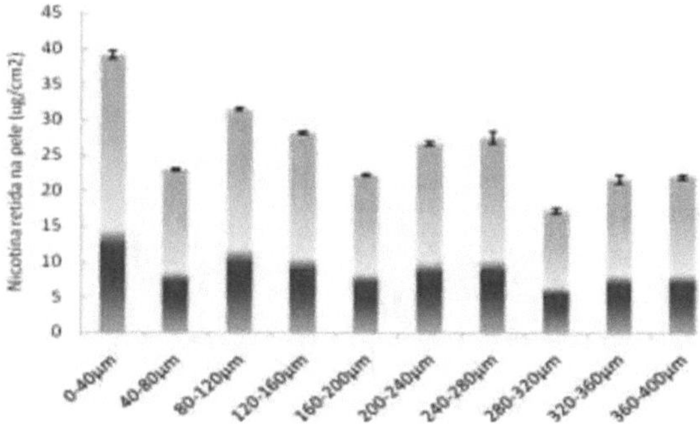

Figura 23. Amounts of nicotine retained in the different layers of pig ear skin using the VDC method in a static system, after 12 hours of permeation, with bars representing the standard deviation (n = 3).

The results obtained with the mapping technique were differentiated into 3 columns: EC (nicotine values found from 0 to 80 µm), EP+D (nicotine values found in the layers from 80 to 400 µm) and total skin (sum of nicotine values found from 0 to 400 µm) with the aim of favoring comparison with the conventional skin retention technique and the results of this comparison are shown in **Figure 24.**

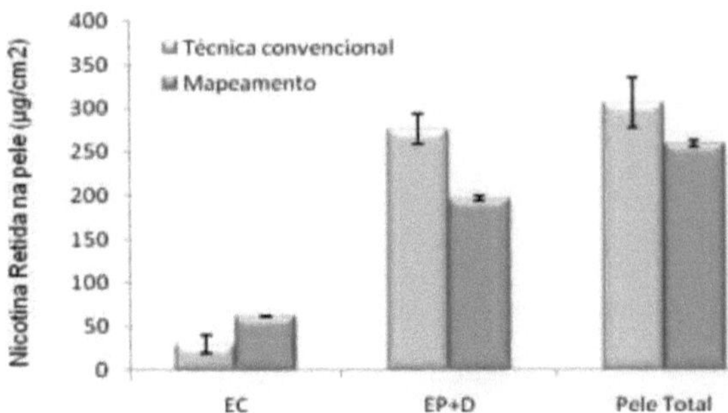

Figura 24. Amounts of nicotine retained in the different layers of pig ear skin (EC and EP+D) using the conventional *tape stripping and* skin retention method with n= 5 and the depth mapping method (skin thickness at 400 µm) with n= 3, both in VDC in a static system, after 12 hours of permeation with the bars representing the standard deviation.

5. DISCUSSION

The validation of the analytical methodology for nicotine by High Performance Liquid Chromatography was carried out in accordance with the guidelines established in Resolution - RE No. 899 of May 29, 2003 of the National Health Surveillance Agency. The parameters of linearity, specificity, selectivity, precision, accuracy, limit of detection, limit of quantification and robustness of the methodology were determined.

At alkaline pH, there is a high possibility of nicotine interacting strongly with the silanol residues of the stationary phases of chromatographic columns, since in this condition 25% of the molecules are in the neutral form (free base). These interactions can lead to chromatograms with broad, tailed peaks (CIOLINO *et al.*, 1999).

To overcome this problem and improve the symmetry of the nicotine peak, Ciolino *et al.* (1999) used a deactivated reserve phase by adding triethylamine to the mobile phase. Pereira *et al.* (2001), in this same situation, opted for the use of diethylamine, which favored good results, such as peak symmetry, due to the competition that occurs between diethylamine and nicotine for the residual silanol groups of the silica present in the chromatographic column.

In the present work, the mobile phase was developed according to Pereira *et al.* (2001) and showed good elution results, with a retention time of around 3 minutes and peak symmetry (**Figure 11**).

The method's specificity and selectivity test was carried out using solutions of possible interferents and compared with the nicotine retention time. As can be seen in **Figures 11** (**A** and **B**), there were no interfering results for this methodology.

The linearity of the analytical curve shown in **Figure 12** and **Table 1** showed a linear correlation coefficient of 0.999. No concentration showed a coefficient of variation greater than 8%, which is in accordance with the parameters established by RE No. 899 of May 29, 2003 of the National Health Surveillance Agency.

The intra- and inter-assay precision and accuracy shown in **Table 2** demonstrate a maximum coefficient of variation of 3.4% and accuracy of over 95.8%. The lower limit of quantification and lower limit of detection of the analytical methodology were determined to be 0.1 and 0.05 μg/mL, respectively, which were below the nicotine concentrations found in the release, permeation and skin retention samples.

The robustness of the analytical methodology evaluated by comparing the nicotine peak areas of the standard solution analyzed before and after varying the oven temperature by± 1°C, varying the mobile phase by 0.5% and varying the batch of the chromatographic column, showed no deviations greater than 10%, indicating that the proposed method for nicotine quantification is a robust analytical method (**Table 3**).

The results found are in line with scientific literature for nicotine quantification by high performance liquid chromatography.

Pereira *et al.* (2001) demonstrated analytical validation for nicotine in CLAE, obtaining linearity between 50 and 5,000 ng/mL with a coefficient of variation of less than 5%, using an RP 18- Select B column and reading at 254 nm.

The apparatus of the foot on disk method (FDA), as well as VDC in a static system and with continuous flow, were validated and the results presented in **Table 4.** It was possible to verify the reproducibility of the factors evaluated, with a coefficient of variation of less than 5%. The linearity of the pumping flow ratio of the receiving medium was shown to be linear with $R^2 = 0.998$. These results helped in choosing the pumping flow of the receiving medium for the following skin release and permeation tests using VDC with continuous flow.

Among the physicochemical tests applied to pharmaceutical forms, release is undoubtedly the most important in assessing the ability of the pharmaceutical form to release its active ingredient (ABDOU, 1995). *In* this way, *in vitro* release tests are one of the essential tools for evaluating the biopharmacotechnical properties of formulations. They also provide useful information for research and development, production and quality control.

In pharmacotechnical development, they enable the evaluation of new formulations, stability checks and *in vitro and in vivo* correlation studies. During the production and quality control phase, these tests make it possible to detect manufacturing deviations, product uniformity and batch-to-batch reproducibility (MARQUES & BROWN, 2002). For drugs that do not have an official monograph, there is a need to develop release tests that can predict their *in vivo* behavior.

The evaluation of the drug release profile (percentage of dissolved drug *versus* time) in different media is recommended to support the development of the release methodology (MANADAS *et al.*, 2002). However, many factors have a strong impact on the variability of drug release tests, so the influence of three important factors in this context was evaluated: (i) composition of the release media, (ii) agitation of the release medium and (iii) batches of the drug (MANADAS *et al.*, 2002).

One of the parameters with the greatest impact on the variability of release tests may be the composition of the receptor medium. To assess the influence of the composition of the receptor medium on nicotine release, different media were tested, including PBS pH 7.4 (± 0.2) 0.01 M phosphate buffer, deionized water and 0,.025 N HCl. As shown in **Figure 14**, the receptor medium that promoted the highest nicotine release rates was PBS phosphate buffer pH 7.4 (± 0.2) 0.01M, showing significant differences at 8 hours when compared to the acidic medium (HCl 0.025 N) and the aqueous medium. In view of the results, phosphate buffer was selected as the receptor medium for the next *in vitro* release and permeation tests.

These results are directly related to the physicochemical characteristics of nicotine, since the absorption of nicotine through membranes depends on pH. If the pH is acidic, nicotine is ionized and does not easily pass through membranes, whereas at physiological pH (pH~ 7.4), 31% of nicotine is not ionized and passes easily through membranes.

Other factors evaluated in the variability of the nicotine release tests were the stirring speed of the receptor medium (**Figure 15**) and different batches of the drug NiQuitin™ 78mg (**Figure 16**). The results shown in **Figure 15** and **Table 5** indicate that the speeds of 50, 75 and 300 rpm were similar. Therefore, the speeds of 50 and 300 rpm were selected for the powder on disk (FDA) and VDC methods respectively, for the following *in vitro* release and skin permeation tests.

Skoug *et al.* (1996), in a discussion on methodologies for drug dissolution tests, suggested typical values for stirring speed of 50 rpm when using paddles and 100 rpm when using baskets, however, stirring values other than these can be accepted with due justification.

The comparison of drug release profiles through the pharmaceutical form is useful in cases where you want to know the behavior of two products before submitting them to relative bioavailability/bioequivalence tests, to exempt the lowest dosages from these studies, in cases of post-registration changes and quality control of medicines (ANVISA Resolution RE No. 310 of September 1, 2004).

The similarity in the release profile of the different batches of the drug NiQuitin™ 78mg (**Figure 16**), demonstrated the pharmaceutical equivalence between the batches that were tested in the permeation and skin retention studies, thus ensuring the absence of variability due to a lack of quality control of the pharmaceutical form.

The evaluation of the effect of the radial diffusion of nicotine in NiQuitin™ adhesives, shown in **Figure 17**, indicates that up to the 8-hour release period, both the whole adhesives and the trimmed adhesives showed values of approximately 100% of the nicotine present in the experimental diffusion area (1.77 $cm^{2)}$. However, at 12 hours it was possible to observe values above this range for the whole adhesive sample, which suggests a possible radial diffusion of the nicotine present in the system by a mechanism not yet evident. For the permeation tests up to 8 hours, no significant difference was found between the trimmed and whole adhesives. Therefore, 8 hours was selected as the maximum release and skin permeation time for the other tests.

Hadgraft *et al.* (1991) suggested that care should be taken when developing release methods for transdermal patches. They identified the influence of edge effect on Franz VDC release for nitroglycerin present in transdermal patches available in the United States. Values of nitroglycerin released from whole patches were around 0.7 times higher when compared to those obtained from trimmed patches. However, this effect was not observed in the skin permeation tests with human skin from the abdominal region, as the presence of the skin was able to control the rate of delivery of the active.

Olivier *et al.* (2003) evaluated the permeation of nicotine in Nicorette transdermal patches®, showing that in permeation periods longer than 28 hours, nicotine in quantities greater than that available per diffusion area was found in the receptor solution and attributed this phenomenon to the edge effect.

As a result, they evaluated the influence of the edge effect on release using different trimming diameters of the transdermal patch, including 1.2 cm^2, 1.8 cm(2)and 2.45 cm^2, in which they observed that the amount of nicotine released from the Nicorette system® per period of time is dependent on the diffusion surface area.

The *in vitro* nicotine release assays for transdermal patches were evaluated and compared using the foot on disk method (FDA), VDC in a static and continuous flow system, which are shown in **Figure 18**.

In terms of the efficiency of nicotine release from transdermal patches, all the methods tested showed results above 80% release up to 8 hours of release.

The accumulated amounts of nicotine released in up to 8 hours were in the order of 5555.21 (±189), 4258.66 (±152) and 5572.0 (±138) µg/cm² for the dust-on-disc method (FDA), and VDC in a static and continuous flow system, respectively. While the release flow values (*J*) calculated from the linear portion of the release curve were 510.5 (±49.8) for FDA, 494.3 (±15.3) for VDC in a static system and 574.8 (±23.2) for VDC in continuous flow.

The values of cumulative amounts µg/cm² in 8 hours, as well as the *J* nicotine, were approximately equal, showing no significant differences when using the statistical methods of analysis based on the non-parametric One-Way ANOVA model ($p < 0.05$).

Innovatively, this research has brought new perspectives to the use of difference (f1) and similarity (f2) factors to evaluate the release profile (**Figure 19**). The data obtained for the different methods for studying *in vitro* release/permeation were compatible with the results obtained when using the One - Way ANOVA statistical model ($p > 0.05$), suggesting that the independent mathematical model f_1 and f_2 can be applied not only to evaluate release profiles obtained through oral solid pharmaceutical forms (FFSO) (RE n° 310 of September 1, 2004), but also for topical/transdermal systems.

Figure 20 shows that the NiQuitinTM nicotine transdermal system has membrane-dependent permeation characteristics, since nicotine values in µg/cm² were found to be 0.8 times higher in 8 hours of permeation with biological membranes, when compared to samples obtained in the absence of a membrane. However, no significant difference was observed in the amount of nicotine permeated at 8 hours for pig ear skin, hairless mouse skin and snake skin moisturized for 24 hours.

Greater deviations between permeation replicates were found for pig ear skin at all collection times. This may be related to the difficulty in controlling the age, sex and diet of the slaughter animals, as well as the preparation of the pig ear skin before the permeation tests, which requires the use of the dermatomization technique. Snakeskin seedlings, as well as hairless mouse skins, were obtained by monitoring the age, weight and sex of the animals, which may have provided considerable reproducibility of the results obtained in the skin permeation tests.

Several scientific studies suggest that pig ear skin is the best substitute for human skin *in in vitro* skin permeation tests. According to Haigh and Smith (1994), pig ear skin is similar to human tissue in terms of hair follicle density.

The use of snake skin as a permeation barrier for drugs has been extensively studied as a model membrane to replace human skin for *in vitro* permeation tests (RIGG, BARRY, 1990; ITOH *et al*, 1990a and b; WIDLER, SIGRIST and GAFNER, 2002), as well as in tests evaluating the effects of a series of skin permeation promoters (WONG *et al.*, 1989; BHATT *et al.*, 1991; HIRVONEN *et al.*, 1991; BHATTACHAR *et al.*, 1992; BUYUKTIMKIN *et al.*, 1993; HIRVONEN *et al.*, 1993; SUH AND JUN, 1996).

In our tests, the ventral regions of the snake skin were selected, as suggested by Haigh *et al.* (1998) who observed that the ventral layer of three different types of snakes and serpents presented itself as a thicker and more resistant layer, as shown in electron microscopy photomicrographs. These findings may be related to the fact that when the snake moves, the ventral layer is always in contact with the surface and this makes it more resistant than the dorsal layer. The dorsal region of the skin of snake moults has been found to be thinner than the ventral region, especially in snakes and serpents (HAIGH *et al.*, 1998).

The pre-treatment of the snakeskin samples, including mechanical removal of the surface layers with adhesive tape and moisturizing at different times, was carried out following the model of Baby et al. They evaluated the interaction of surfactants with *Bothrops jararaca* snake skin seedlings using spectrometric (infrared photoacoustic and Raman spectroscopy) and thermoanalytical (differential scanning calorimetry) techniques. They found that the surfactants sodium dodecyl sulfate, hexadecyl trimethyl ammonium chloride and PEG-12 lauryl ether interacted with the skin only after the surface layers of the tissue were mechanically removed with adhesive tape. These results show that, in addition to the *mesolayer*, the β-layer contributes to the barrier effect of snakeskin seedlings, reducing the permeability of this tissue to other active substances in diffusion studies. The same had already been reported by Itoh et al. (1990a) and Takahashi et al. (1993), who identified in their work that the intermediate or *meso* layer is the main obstacle to the permeability of substances.

In our results, it was possible to observe that the pre-treatment of snake skin at different hydration times had a great influence on nicotine permeation rates. Skins hydrated for 24 hours were approximately 4 times more permeable to nicotine when compared to 48-hour hydration, showing significantly different results ($p < 0.05$) **Table 6**.

Over the decades, much attention has been paid to the penetration of water into the skin. Interestingly, this small polar molecule has a profound influence on the skin's barrier properties. Several studies have shown that moisturizing the skin *in a* water bath prior to *in vitro* permeation tests acts as an enhancer of skin permeation, as it generally becomes more permeable when compared to unmoisturized skin (PONGJANYAKUL et al., 2002; HAIGH et al., 1998; MEGRAB et al., 1995).

It was observed that there was no significant difference in the use of the different animal skins (pig ear, hairless mouse and snake skin previously moisturized for 24 hours) up to 8 hours of permeation. Pig ear skin 80 was therefore selected as the membrane model for the *in vitro* evaluation of nicotine permeation, using the FDA, static VDC and continuous flow methods (**Figure 21**).

The amounts of nicotine permeated in μg/cm^2 of pig ear skin, as well as the flow rate *(J* = μg/cm^{2}h^{-1} *)* up to 8 hours of permeation were significantly lower for the feet-on-disc (FDA) method when compared to the results in VDC in both static and continuous flow systems (**Table 6**). These results may be correlated with the physical structure of the VDC equipment, since it offers an occlusive system, making it difficult for the transdermal *patch to* come into contact with the receiving medium, while the metal sandwich formed by the *transdermal patch holder* being placed submerged in the receiving medium may allow the receiving phase to come into contact with the product, thus reducing contact between the patch and the skin.

The skin retention tests on the different layers of pig ear skin using VDC in a static system and the foot on disk method (FDA) are shown in **Figure 22**. The results show greater retention in the EC when the FDA method was used. This fact can be better understood when analyzed together with the results of retention in the EP + D layers (without stratum corneum), which showed low retention of nicotine in the deeper layers of the skin, suggesting that the use of the FDA method promotes greater retention of nicotine in the skin barrier, not favoring its permeation in the deeper layers and consequently hindering the permeation of the active into the receptor medium. These results may explain the lower permeation flux obtained when the FDA powder method was used.

Analyzing the nicotine retention tests on total skin, i.e. on all the layers of skin, when using the VDC method in a static system, we observed greater retention of the active ingredient in pig ear skin. These results seem to indicate that the greater the retention of the active ingredient in all layers of the skin, especially the deeper layers, the greater its penetration through the skin.

If we take into account the fact that the *in vitro* procedure for studying permeation generally takes place through the diffusion of the drug by concentration gradient through the membrane, it is possible to understand the importance of the active ingredient being present in all layers of the skin, especially the deepest ones, so that penetration through it is more successful.

Mapping drug retention at different skin depths is able to demonstrate the depth of permeation characteristics of a transdermal or topical release system.

Jenning *et al.,* 2000 reported that layers above 100 μm of pig ear skin represent mainly the EC, layers between 100 and 200 μm are represented in greater quantity by the epidermis, while layers between 200 and 500 μm are found basically the epidermis+ viable dermis.

In order to map the depth of nicotine retention in pig ear skin after 12 hours of *in vitro* permeation, the method for assessing retention in successive layers of skin was validated after a permeation study using VDC in a static system. The results obtained are shown in **Figure 23**, and suggest that similar amounts of nicotine are present in every 40 μm of skin, indicating nicotine partitioning in all the skin layers evaluated.

Echevarria *et al.,* 2003 evaluated the skin retention characteristics of mupirocin applied topically to the different layers of pig ear skin after 24 hours of permeation. Using several 40 μm skin sections in a horizontal direction, they found greater accumulation of mupirocin in the skin layers from 40 to 200 μm and a significant decrease in the amount of the active ingredient from 240 μm, remaining constant up to 400 μm.

For a comparative analysis of the retention results obtained by the depth mapping technique with the conventional retention technique, the nicotine values determined in the different layers of the skin were differentiated into 3 columns: EC (nicotine values found between the layers from 0 to 80 μm), EP+D (nicotine values found between the layers from 80 to 400 μm) and total skin (sum of the nicotine values found in the layers from 0 to 400 μm) **Figure 24**.

These results showed nicotine retention values very close to those found with the conventional skin retention technique, with the cumulative amounts of nicotine in total skin showing slightly lower values. These results may be correlated with the fact that in the conventional technique, pig ear skin was dermatomized at 500 μm, while in the mapping technique, horizontal cuts were made up to 400 μm.

6. CONCLUSIONS

The analytical methodology proposed for nicotine quantification after *in vitro* release, permeation and skin retention tests proved to be effective, sensitive, precise, accurate and robust for the purpose proposed.

With the results of nicotine release from transdermal patches, by evaluating different factors in the variability of drug release tests, it was possible to select the most suitable receptor medium and the agitation speed of the receptor medium. In these tests, it was possible to obtain greater reproducibility of analysis and greater nicotine release when using the VDC method in a static system, using alkaline receptor medium, indicating that the specifications laid down in the American Pharmacopoeia do not always guarantee the most suitable methodology for the needs of each test and drug.

Verifying that the permeation results were not variable from batch to batch was of great importance, since pharmaceutical equivalence was demonstrated in the release profile of all the batches selected for the *in vitro* release, permeation and skin retention tests.

The results obtained using the difference (f_1) and similarity (f_2) factors to evaluate the nicotine release profile of transdermal patches were comparable to the results obtained using the non-parametric OneWay ANOVA statistical model, assuming $p > 0.05$. This demonstrated the efficiency of using the independent mathematical model f_1 and f_2 not only to compare the release profiles of oral solid pharmaceutical forms, but also to evaluate the comparative permeation profile of transdermal patches.

The nicotine release tests in the absence of a membrane using VDC, both in a static system and in continuous flow, showed similar results to those obtained with the method indicated by the FDA, both in quantities released in µg/cm^2 and in flow *(J)* up to 8 hours. This indicates that the use of the VDC and FDA methods for *in vitro* drug release tests on transdermal patches can be interchangeable.

The results of nicotine permeation through biological membranes indicated that the release of nicotine present in NiQuitin™ transdermal patches is membrane-dependent. Hairless mouse skin, as well as snake seedling skin, showed greater reproducibility when compared to pig ear skin, indicating that controlling the age, sex and feeding of the animals used may be significant factors in the repeatability of the results. However, the coefficient of variation values presented are in line with the parameters stipulated in the SCCP guidelines, where the coefficient of variation must be less than 30% for an experiment containing n = 6 (SCCP, 2006).

Skin retention tests, both by the conventional *tape stripping* method and by depth mapping, have demonstrated the importance of nicotine partitioning into all layers of the skin to favor permeation through the skin.

The results of this project may indicate the use of VDC in a static system and with continuous flow as satisfactory methods for *in vitro* tests of the release and skin permeation of transdermal drugs. They can be applied both in research into the development of formulations and in quality control and pharmaceutical equivalence studies for generic drugs administered transdermally.

The data obtained in this study could help in the discussions around generic drugs in Brazil, influencing the guidelines for Pharmaceutical Equivalence and Quality Control tests of transdermal drugs, both for the standardization of the apparatus model to be used and also in the proposition of mathematical models for comparing release profiles.

BIBLIOGRAPHIC REFERENCE

1. ABDOU H. M. Dissolution, Bioavailability & Bioequivalence. Easton: ***Mack Publishing Company*** pg 544, 1989.

2. ABRAHAM M.K., CHADHA H.S., MITCHELL R.C. The factors that influence skin penetration of solutes. ***J. Pharmacol***., 47:8-16, 1995.

3. ABUZARUR-ALOUL, R.; GJELLAN K.; SJOLUND M.; LOFQVIST M. GRADDNER. C. Critical dissolution test of oral systems based on statistically designed experiments. I: Screening of critical fluids and in vivo/in vivo modeling of extended release coated spheres. ***Drug Dev. Ind. Pharm***., 23(8):749-760, 1997.

4. AIACHE, J. M. Apparatus for studying the dissolution speed of drugs from non-oral forms. In: Arancibia, A. Pezoa, R. eds. Bioavailability of Medicines: ***International Symposium I. Santiago*** : Editorial Universitària, pp.125149, 1992.

5. AIACHE, M.; CHANET, L.; BEYSSAC, E; HAIGER, M.J. In vitro permeation of progesterone from a gel through the shed skin of three different snake species. ***Int. J. . Pharm.,*** 170:151-156, 1998.

6. ALIBERTI, A. L. M., DE QUEIROZ, A. C., PRAÇA, F. S. G., ELOY, J.O., BENTLEY, M. V. L. B., MEDINA, W. S. G. Ketoprofen Microemulsion for Improved Skin Delivery and In Vivo Anti-inflammatory Effect. ***AAPS PHARMSCITECH***, 1-9, 2017.

7. ALLEN JR., LOYD V. Pharmaceutical forms and drug delivery systems / LOYD V. ALLEN JR., NICHOLAS G. POPOVICH, HOWARD C ANSEL; transl. Elenara Lemos Senna, 8 ed.

8. ANSEL C. HOWARD, NICHOLAS G. POPOVICH AND LOYD V. Pharmaceutical Dosage forms and Drug Delivery Systems - 6th Ed. Williams & Wilkins, Baltimore, USA, 2000.

9. ASCENO, A.; PINHO, S.; AULETERIO, C.; PRAÇA, F.S.G; OLIVEIRA, H.; BENTLEY, MARIA VITÓRIA LOPES BADRA; SANTOS, C.; SILVA, O.; SIMOES, S. Lycopene from Tomatoes: Vesicular Nanocarrier Formulations for Dermal Delivery. ***J. .Agric. and Food Chem.***, 61:7284-7293, 2013.

10. ASCENO, A.; SARA RAPOSO; CATIA BATISTA; PEDRO CARDOSO; TIAGO MENDES; PRAÇA, F.S.G.; BENTLEY, MARIA VITÓRIA L.B.; SIMOES, S.

Development, characterization, and skin delivery studies of related ultradeformable vesicles: transfersomes, ethosomes, and transethosomes. ***Int. J. Nanomed.,*** 10:5837-5851, 2015.

11. ASCENSO, ANDREIA ; SALGADO, ANA ; EULETÉRIO, CARLA ; PRAÇA, FABiOLA GARCIA ; BENTLEY, MARIA VITÓRIA LOPES BADRA ; MARQUES, HELENA C. ; OLIVEIRA, HELENA ; SANTOS, CONCEIÇÂO ; SIMOES, SANDRA . In vitro and in vivo topical delivery studies of tretinoin-loaded ultradeformable vesicles. ***Eur. J. Pharm. Biopharm.,*** 88:48-55, 2014.

12. ASSOCIAÇÂO BRASILEIRA DE NORMAS TECNICAS, ***NBR 6023***: informaçôes e documentaçôes, referencias:elaboração. Rio de Janeiro, 2002.

13. AYMAN EL-KATTAN, CHARLES S. ASBILL AND SAM HAIDAR. Transdermal testing: practical aspects and methods. ***PSTT***, 3 (12), 2000.

14. BABY A. R, CARLOS ALBERTO HAROUTIOUNIAN-FILHO, FERNANDA DAUD SARRUF, CARLOS ROBERTO TAVANTE-JÛNIOR, CLAUDINÉIA APARECIDA SALES DE OLIVEIRA PINTO, VIVIAN ZAGUE, ELIZABETH PINHEIRO GOMES ARÊAS, TELMA MARY KANEKO, MARIA VALÉRIA ROBLES VELASCO. Stability and in vitro skin penetration study of rutin in a cosmetic emulsion using an alternative biomembrane model. ***Braz. J. Pharm. Sc.,*** 44(2):Apr./Jun., 2008.

15. BABY AR, LACERDA ACL, KAWANO Y, VELASCO MVR, LOPES OS, KANEKO TM PAS-FTIR and FT-Raman qualitative characterization of sodium dodecyl sulfate interaction with an alternative stratum corneum model membrane. ***Pharmazie,*** 62(10):727-731, 2007.

16. BABY AR, LACERDA ACL, KAWANO Y, VELASCO MVR, LOPES OS, KANEKO TM. Evaluation of the interaction of surfactants with stratum corneum model membrane from Bothrops jararaca by DSC. ***Int. J. Pharm***., v.317, 1: 7-9, 2006a.

17. BABY AR, LACERDA ACL, KAWANO Y, VELASCO MVR, LOPES OS, KANEKO TM Spectroscopic studies of stratum corneum model membrane from Bothrops jararaca treated with cationic surfactant. ***Colloid. Surf. B Biointer***.,50(1):61-65, 2006b.

18. BANAKAR, U.V. Pharmaceutical Dissolution Testing. New York, ***Marcel Dekker Inc***, pp 437, 1992.

19. BARBERO, A.M, FRASCH, H.F. Pig and guinea pig skin as surrogates for human in vitro penetration studies: A quantitative review. ***Toxicol Vitr***., 23(1):1-13, 2009.

20. BARRY B.W, Dermatological Formulation. Percutaneous absorption. ***Drug and Pharm. Sci.***,50, p.480, 1983.

21. BENOWITZ NL. Nicotine safety and toxicity. New York: Oxford ***University Press***; 1998.

22. BENTLEY, M.V., VIANNA, R. F., COLLETT J., Characterization of the Influence of some Cyclodextrins on the Stratum Corneum from the Hairless Mouse. ***J. Pharm. Pharmacol***. 49 (4):397-402, 1997.

23. BHATT, P.P., RYTTING, J.H., TOPP, E.M. Influence of azone and lauryl alcohol on the transport of acetaminophen and ibuprofen through shed snake skin. ***Int. J. Pharm***. 72, 219-226, 1991.

24. BHATTACHAR, S.N., RYTTING, J.H., ITOH, T., NISHIHATA, T. The effects of complexation with hydrogenated phospholipid on the transport of salicylic acid, diclofenac and indomethacin

across snake stratum corneum. ***Int. J. Pharm***. 79:263271, 1992.

25. BRAZIL, National Health Surveillance Agency ***RE No. 310*** of September 1, 2004. Guide for conducting pharmaceutical equivalence tests with dissolution profile for FFSO.

26. BRAZIL, National Health Surveillance Agency ***RE No. 893*** of May 29, 2003. Guide to making changes, additions and notifications after drug registration.

27. BRAZIL. National Health Surveillance Agency ***RE n.899*** of May 29, 2003. Determines the publication of the "Guide to the validation of analytical and bioanalytical methods".

28. BRITISH PHARMACOPEIA 2009. London v. 2: Her Majesty's Stationery Office.

29. BRONAUGH, R.L.; STEWART, R.F. Methods for in vitro percutaneous absorption studies III: hydrophobic compounds. ***J. Pharm. Sci.***, 73: 1255-1258, 1985.

30. BU0201/02- NiQuitin™ package leaflet

31. BUYUKTIMKIN, S., BUYUKTIMKIN, N., RYTTING, J.H. Synthesis and enhancing effect of 2-(N,N-dimethylamino) propionate on the transepidermal delivery of indomethacin, clonidine and hydrocortisone. ***Pharm. Res.*** 10:1632-1637,1993.

32. CAMPOS, P. M.; PRAÇA, F.S.G.; BENTLEY, MARIA VITÓRIA L.B.. Quantification of lipoic acid from skin samples by HPLC using ultraviolet, electrochemical and evaporative light scattering detectors. ***J. Chrom. B***, 1:1-20, 2015.

33. CHOWDARY, K.P.R., RAJYALAKSHMI Y. Dissolution rate in modern pharmacy. ***East Pharm. New Delhi***, 30 (350):51-54, 1987.

34. CIOLINO LA, TURNER JA, MCCAULEY HA, SMALLWOOD AW, YI TYJ. Optimization study for the reversed-phase ion pair liquid chromatographic determination of nicotine in commercial tobacco products. ***J Chrom. A***., 852(2): 451463, 1999.

35. COLDMAN, M.F., POULSEN, B.F., HIGUCHI, T. Enhancement of percutaneous absorption by the use of volatile: nonvolatile systems as vehicles. ***J. Pharm. Sci***. 58:1098-1102, 1969.

36. DEPIERI, L.V., PRAÇA, F.S., CAMPOS, P.M., BENTLEY, M.V. Advances in the bioanalytical study of drug delivery across the skin. ***Ther Deliv***. 6(5):571-94, 2015.

37. ECHEVARRiA L, BLANCO-PRiETO MJ, CAMPANERO MA, SANTOYO S, YGARTUA P. Development and validation of a liquid chromatographic method for in vitro mupirocin quantification in both skin layers and percutaneous penetration studies. ***J Chrom. B*** Analyt Technol Biomed Life Sci. 5;796(2):233-41,2003.

38. EL TAYAR, N.; RUEY-SHIUAM, T.; TESYA, B.; CARUPT, P. A. Percutaneous of drugs: A quantitative structure-permeability relationship study. **J. Pharm. Sci.**, 80:744749, 1991.

39. ELIAS, P.M. Structure and function of the Stratum Corneum extracellular matrix. ***J Invest***

Dermatol,132(9):2131 -3, 2013.

40. ELVIRA ESCRIBANO, ANA CRISTINA CALPENA, JOSEP QUERALT, ROSSEND OBACH AND JOSE DOMÉNECH. Assessment of diclofenac permeation with different formulations: anti-inflammatory study of a selected formula. **Eur. J. Pharm. Sci.,**19 (4):203-210, 2003.

41. ESTRACANHOLLI, E.A.; PRAÇA, F.S.G.; CINTRA, A. B.; Maria Bernadete Riemma Pierre; Lara, Marilisa Guimaraes. Liquid Crystalline Systems for Transdermal Delivery of Celecoxib: In Vitro Drug Release and Skin Permeation Studies. ***AAPS PharmSciTech***, 1:1, 2014.

42. EUROPEAN PHARMACOPOEIA 2004, 5th Ed. v.2 Council of Europe: France, Strasbourg.

43. FANG, J.Y.; WU P.C.; HUANG Y.B.; TSAI Y.H. In vitro permeation study of capsaicin and its synthetic derivates from ointment bases using various skin types. ***In. J. Pharm.,*** 126:119-128, 1995.

44. FANT V. R.; LUCY L. O. D.; JACK E. H. Nicotine replacement therapy. ***Primary Care: Clinics in Office Practice***, 26(3):633-652, 1999.

45. FARE H.M.; ZATZ J.L. Measurement of drug release from topical gels using two types of apparatus. ***Pharm. Tech.*** 19(1):52-58, 1995.

46. AMERICAN PHARMACOPE -USP 29, Rockville, 2006.

47. EUROPEAN PHARMCOPE - 4th Ed. France, 2002.

48. FDA - Guidance for industry: SUPAC-SS Nonsterile Semisolid Dosage forms. Scale- up and Post approval changes: Chemistry, manufacturing and controls: in vitro release testing and in vivo Bioequivalence Documentation , may 1997.

49. FDA - Guidelines for dissolution testing of solid oral products. Drug Inf. J. Philadelphia, 30:1071-1784, 1996.

50. FDA. Guidance for industry: SUPAC-SS Nonsterile semisolids dosage forms. Scale- up and post approval changes: chemistry, manufacturing and controls: in vitro release testing and in vivo bioequivalence documentation. 1999.

51. FELDMANN, R.J., MAIBACH, H.I.Regional variation in percutaneous penetration of 14C cortisol in man. ***J Invest Dermatol.*** ,48(2):181-3, 1967.

52. FISCHMEISTER, I., HELLGREN, L., VINCENT, J. Infrared spectroscopy for tracing of topically applied ointment vehicles and active substances on healthy skin. ***Arch Dermatol Res***, 253: 63-69, 1975.

53. FLEEKER, C., WONG, O., RYTTING, J.H. Facilitated transport of basic and acidic drugs in solutions through snake skin by a new enhancer-dodecyl N,N- dimethylamino acetate. ***Pharm. Res.*** 6: 443-448, 1989.

54. FLYNN C.L.; SHAH V.P.; TENJARLA S.N. et. al. Assessment of value and applications of in

vitro testing of topical dermatological drug products. ***Pharm. Res***. 16: 1325-1330, 1999.

55. FOULDS J, STAPLETON J, HAYWARD M, RUSSELL MAH, FEYERABEND C, FLEMING T, et al. Transdermal nicotine patches with low-intensity support to aid smoking cessation in outpatients in a general hospital. ***Arc. Fam. Med,*** 2:417-23, 1993.

56. FRANZ J.T. Percutaneous absorption. On the relevance of in vitro data. ***J. Invest. Dermatol***., 64:190-195, 1975.

57. FU LU, M., LEE, D., SUBBA RAO, G. Percutaneous absorption enhancement of leuprolide. ***Pharm. Res***. 9:1575-1579, 1992.

58. GAO S, SINGH J. Effect of oleic acid/ethanol and oleic/propylene glycol on the in vitro percutaneous absorption of 5-fluorouracil and tamoxifen and the macroscopic barrier property of porcine epidermis. ***Int. J. Pharm.,*** 165: 45-55, 1998.

59. GARCIA F. S.; TEDESCO A. C.; COLLETT J.H.; BENTLEY M. L.V. Topical Delivery System for ZnPcSO4 based on Liquid Crystalline phases for use in PDT of skin Cancer. Controlled Release Society - 31 st *Annual Meeting and Exposition of the Controlled Release Society,*1:320-320, 2004.

60. GORDON L. FLYNN. Fundamental Concepts of in vitro Release. AAPS-FDA Workshop on Assessment of value applications of in vitro release testing of topical dermatological drug products, sept 1997.

61. GORROD, J. W.; JACOB III, P. Analytical determination of nicotine and related compounds and their metabolites. ***Elsevier Science***, 772, 1999.

62. GUIDELINES Mental and Behavioural Disorders. Clinical descriptions and diagnostic guideliness, 1992.

63. HADGRAFT J, LEWIS D, BEUTNER D AND WOLFF MH. "In vitro assessments of transdermal devices containing nytroglycerin." ***Int. J. Pharm.,*** (73):125-130, 1991.

64. HADGRAFT, J. Skin deep. ***Eur. J. Pharm. Biopharm***., 58(2):291-299, 2004.

65. HADGRAFT, J. Skin, the final frontier. ***Int. J. Pharm***., 224(1/2):1-18, 2001.

66. HADGRAFT, J.; RIDOUT, G. Development of model membranes for percutaneous absorption measurements. I. Isopropyl myristate***. Int. J. Pharm***., 39(1/2):149-156, 1987.

67. HADGRAFT, J.W., SOMERS G. F. PERCUTANEOUS ABSORPTION ***J. Pharm. Pharmacol.*** 8 (1): 625-634, 1956.

68. HAIGH JM, SMITHEW EW 1994. The selection of natural and synthetic membranes for in vitro diffusion experiments***. Eur. J. Pharm. Sci***., 2 (5/6): 311-330, 1994.

69. HAIGH, J.M.; BEYSSAC, E.; CHANET, L.; AIACHE, J.-M. In vitro permeation of progesterone from a gel through the shed snake skin of three different species. ***Int. J.Pharm.,*** 170(2):151-156,

1998.

70. HANSON RESEARCH COORPORATION - www.hansonresearch.com

71. HIGUCHI, W. I., HIGUCHI T. Theoretical analysis of diffusional movement through heterogeneous barriers. ***J. Pharm. Sci.***, 49: 598-606, 1960.

72. HIRVONEN, J., RYTTING, J.H., PARONEN, P., URTTI, A. Dodecyl N,N- dimethylamino acetate and Azone enhance drug penetration across human, snake and rabbit skin. ***Pharm. Res.*** 8:933-937, 1991.

73. HUGHES JR, GOLDSTEIN MG, HURT RD, SHIFFMAN S. Recent advances in the pharmacotherapy of smoking. ***JAMA***;281(1):72-6, 1999.

74. ITOH T, XIA J, MAGAVI R, NISHIHATA T, RYTTING JH. Use of shed snake skin as a model membrane for in vitro percutaneous penetration studies: comparison with human skin. ***Pharm. Res.***, 7(10):1042-1047, 1990a.

75. ITOH T, MAGAVI R, CASADY RL, NIISHIHATA T, RYTTING JH. A method to predict the percutaneous permeability of various compounds: shed snake skin as a model membrane. ***Pharm. Res.***, 7(12):1302-1306, 1990b.

76. J. KEMKEN, A. ZIEGLER, B. W. MIILLER, ***J. Pharm. Pharmacol.***, 43: 679, 1991.

77. JENNING V, GYSLER A, SCHAFER-KORTING M, GOHLA S H. Vitamin A loaded solid lipid nanoparticles for topical use: occlusive properties and drug targeting to the upper skin. **Eur. *J. Pharm. Biopharm***, 49:211-218, 2000.

78. JIA-YOU FANG, TSONG-LONG HWANG, CHIA-LANG FANG AND HSIEN-CHIH CHIU. In vitro and in vivo evaluations of the efficacy and safety of skin permeation enhancers using flurbiprofen as a model drug . ***Int. J. Pharm.***, 255 (l-2):153-166, 2003.

79. JORENBY DE, HATSUKAMI DK, SMITH SS, FIORE MC, ALLEN S, JENSEN J, et al. Characterization of tobacco withdrawal symptoms: transdermal nicotine reduces hunger and weight gain. ***Psychopharmacol.,*** 128(2):130-138, 1996.

80. JORGENSEN, E. D.; BHAGWAT, D. Development of dissolution tests for oral extended-release products. ***PSTT***, 1(3):128-135, 1998.

81. JUNQUEIRA L.C., CARNEIRO J. Histologia Bàsica. Translation of Histologia Bàsica, 8th Ed. Editora Guanabara Koogan - Rio de Janeiro, 1995.

82. LOFFLER H, DREHER F, MAIBACH HI. Stratum corneum adhesive tape stripping: influence of anatomical site, application pressure, duration and removal. ***Br J Dermatol***, 151:746-752, 2004.

83. LOPES B. L.; COLLET J.H. BENTLEY M.V.L.B. Topical delivery of cyclosporin A: an in vitro study using monoolein as a penetration enhancer ***Eur. J. Pharm. Biopharm.***, 60(1):25-30, 2005.

84. LOPES, R.F.V.; BENTLEY, M.V.L.; DELGADO-CHARRO, M.B.; GUY, R.H. Iontophoretic delivery of 5-aminolevulinic acid (ALA): effect of pH. ***Pharm. Res.***, 18:311-315, 2001.

85. M. AKAZAWA, T. ITOH, K. MASAK, B.T. NGHIEM, N. TSUZUKI, R. KONISHI, T. HIGUCHI. ***Int. J. Pharm***, 50,53, 1989.

86. MANADAS R.; PINA M. EM; VEIGA F. In vitro dissolution in the prediction of oral absorption of drugs in modified release pharmaceutical forms. ***Rev. Bràs. Cien. Farm***., 38(4):375-399, 2002.

87. MARCOLONGO R. & STORPIRTIS S. Drug dissolution: fundamentals, applications, regulatory aspects and perspectives in the pharmaceutical field. In press. Master's Thesis, FCF-USP, 2003.

88. MARQUES, M.R.C.; BROWN, W. Development and validation of dissolution methods for oral solid pharmaceutical forms. ***Rev. Anal***., 1:48-51, 2002.

89. MEGRAB NA, WILLIAMS AC, BARRY BW. Estradiol permeation across human skin, silastic and snake skin membranes: the effects of ethanol/water cosolvent systems. ***Int. J. Pharm***. 116(1):101-112, 1995.

90. NERNST, W. Theorie der Reaktionsgeschwindigkeit in heterogenen Systemen. Z. ***Phys. Chem.*** 47, 52-55, 1904.

91. NOYES A.A.; WITHNEY, W.R.; The rate of solution of solid substances in their own solutions. ***J. Am. Chem. Soc.*** 19:930-934, 1897.

92. NUNES, R.S., AZEVEDO, J.R., VASCONCELOS, A.P., PEREIRA, N.L. Study of the standardization of snake skin - Boa constrictor - as a stratum corneum model for drug permeation. ***Sci plena***. 1(7):171-5, 2005.

93. OECD. Guideline for the testing of chemicals, n°428. ***Skin Absorption: In vitro Method***, Paris, France, 2004.

94. OLIVIER J.C, RABOUAN S., COUET W., In vitro comparative studies of two marketed transdermal nicotine delivery systems: Nicopatch and Nicorette. ***Int. J. Pharm.,*** 252, 133-140, 2003.

95. PACKER, K.J., SELLWOOD, T.C. Proton magnetic resonance studies of hydrated stratum corneum part 1. Spin-lattice and transverse relaxation. ***J. Chem. Soc.*** Faraday Trans II, 74: 1579-1591, 1978.

96. PEREIRA G. R.; COLLET, J.H.; BENTLEY, M.V.L. B. Effect of GMO\ Propyleneglycol systems on in vitro nicotine's skin permeation. ***Eur. J. Pharm. Sci.,*** 13(1):1131-132, 2001.

97. PETRILLI, R.; ELOY, J.O.; PRAÇA, F.S.G. ; CIAMPO, J.O. ; FANTINI, M.C.A; FONSECA, M.J. ; BENTLEY, MARIA VITÓRIA L.B. Liquid Crystalline Nanodispersions Functionalized with Cell-Penetrating Peptides for Topical Delivery of Short-Interfering RNAs: A Proposal for Silencing a Pro-Inflammatory Cytokine in Cutaneous Diseases. ***J. Biom. Nanotech***, 12:1063-1075, 2016.

98. PETRILLI, R.; PRAÇA, F.S.G.; ALINE CAROLLO; MEDINA, W. S. G.; OLIVEIRA, K. T.; FANTINI, M. C. A.; NEVES, M. G. P. M.; CAVALEIRO, J. A. S.; SERRA, O. A.; IAMAMOTO, Y.; BENTLEY, MARIA VITÓRIA LOPES BADRA . Nanoparticles of lyotropic liquid crystals: a novel strategy for the topical delivery of a chlorine derivative for photodynamic therapy of skin cancer. ***Current Nanoscience***, 9: 434441, 2013.

99. PHARMACOPEIAL FORUM 2009. Topical and transdermal drug products - Products quality tests, vol 35 (3) May-June, 2009.

100. PONGJANYAKUL T, PRAKONGPAN S, PANOMSUK S, PUTTIPIPATKHACHORN S, PRIPREM A. Shed king cobra and cobra skins as model membranes for in vitro nicotine permeation studies. ***J. Pharm. Pharmacol***., 54 (10): 1345-1350, 2002.

101. PONGJANYAKUL, T.; PRAKONGPAN, S.; PRIPREM, A. Permeation studies comparing cobra skin with human skin using nicotine trandermal patches. ***Drug Dev. Ind. Pharm.,*** 26:635-642, 2000.

102. PRAÇA, F. S. G.; BENTLEY, M. V. L. B. ; LARA, M. G. ; PIERRE, M. B. R. Celecoxib determination in different layers of skin by a newly developed and validated HPLC-UV method. BMC. ***Biom. Chrom***., 25(11):1237-44, 2011.

103. PRAÇA, F. S. G.; MEDINA, W. S. G. ; PETRILLI, R. ; BENTLEY, MARIA VITÓRIA LOPES BADRA . Liquid Crystal Nanodispersions Enable the Cutaneous Delivery of Photosensitizer for Topical PDT: Fluorescence Microscopy Study of Skin Penetration. ***Current Nanoscience***, 8:535-540, 2012.

104. RIBANI M. Validation of chromatographic and electrophoretic methods. ***Quimica Nova***, 27(5):771-780, 2004.

105. RICHARD GH AND JONATHAN HADGRAFF. ***J. Control. Release*** 4: 237-251. 1987.

106. RIGG, P.C.; BARRY, B.W. Shed snake skin and hairless mouse skin as a model membrane for human skin during permeation studies. ***J. Invest. Dermatol***., 94(2):235-240, 1990.

107. RIGOTTI NA, ARNSTEN JH, MCKOOL KM, WOOD-REID KM, SINGER DE, PASTERNAK RC. The use of nicotine-replacement therapy by hospitalized smokers. ***Am. J. Prev. Med.*** 17(4):255-259, 1999.

108. ROSEMBERG, J. Nicotine: Universal Drug. Sao Paulo: SES/CVE, 174 p. 3, 2003.

109. ROTHMAN, S. The principles of percutaneous absorptionJ. ***Lab. Clin. Med.***, 28p. 1305,1943.

110. ROUSSEL G, ROCHE D, MOMAS I, BRAHIMI N, CALLAIS F, LEQUANG NT, ET AL. Usefulness of markers in managing tobacco withdrawal. ***Pathol. Biol.,*** 45(6):467- 471, 1997.

111. SARA ZORIN, FREDRIK KUYLENSTIERNA and HANS THULIN, In vitro test of Nicotine's permeability through human skin. Risk evaluation and Safety Aspects. ***Ann. Occup. Hyg,*** 43(6):405-413, 1999.

112. SARTORELLI P.; ANDERSEN H.R.; ANGERER J.; CORISH J.; DREXLER H.; GOEN T.; GRIFFIN P.; HOTCHKISS S.A.M.; LARESE F.; MONTOMOLI L.; PERKINS J., SCHMELZ M.; VAN de SANDT J.; WILLIAMS F. Percutaneous penetration studies for risk assessment. ***Env. Toxicol. Pharmacol.***, 8:133-152, 2000.

113. SAUL SHIFFMAN; STUART FERGUSON; STEPHEN HELLEBUSCH. Physician's counseling of patients when prescribing nicotine replacement therapy. ***Addictive Behaviors***, 32(4):728-739, 2007.

114. SCCP 0970/06. Opinion on Basic Criteria for the In vitro assessment of dermal absorption of cosmetic ingredients. Scientific Committee on consumer Products, Adopted by the SCCP, 28 march, 2006.

115. SCHOMOOK F.P.; MEINGASSNER J.G.; BILLICH A. Comparison of human skin or epidermis models with humana skin and animal skin in vitro percutaneous absorption. ***Int. J. Pharm.***, 215: 51-56, 2001.

116. SHAH P VINOD, JEROMES S ELKINS AND ROGER L WILLIAMS. Evaluation of the test system used for in vitro release of drugs for topical dermatological drug products. ***Pharm. Dev. Technol.,*** 4:377-385, 1999.

117. SHAH V.P.; ELKINS J. In vitro release from glucocorticosteroid ointments. ***J. Pharm. Sc***., 84:1139-1140, 1995.

118. SHAH V.P.; ELKINS J.S.; WILLIAMS R.L. Evaluation of the test system used for in vitro release of drugs from topical dermatological drug products. ***Pharm. Develop. Technol.,*** 377-385, 1994.

119. SHIFFMAN S, GITCHELL J, PINNEY JM, BURTON SL, KEMPER KE, LARA EA. Public health benefit of over-the-counter nicotine medications. ***Tobacco Control*** 6(4):306-10, 1997.

120. SIEWERT M.; DRESSMAN J.; BROWN C.; SHAH V.P. FIP/AAPS Guidlines for dissolution in vitro release testing of novel/special dosage forms. ***Dissol. Tech.,*** 10(1):6-15, 2003.

121. SINKO PATRICK J. MARTIN. Fisico farmacia e ciencias farmaceuticas/Patrick J. Sinko; traduçao George Gonzales Ortega, et al. - 5 ed. Porto Alegre: Artmed, 2008.

122. SKOUG J.W.; HALSTEAD G.W.; THEIS D.L.; FFREEMAN J.E.; FAGAN D.T.; ROHRS B.R. Strategy for the development and validation of Dissolution tests for solid oral dosage forms. ***Pharm. Technol.,*** 58-72, 1996.

123. SMITH, D.E., LEWIS, Y.S. PREPARATION AND EFFECTS OF AN ANTI-MAST CELL SERUM. ***J Exp Med***. 31;113(4):683-92,1961.

124. STAPLETON J, RUSSELL M, FEYRABEND C, WISEMAN S, et al. Dose effects and predictors of outcome in a randomized trial of transdermal nicotine patches in general practice. ***Addict.*** 90:31-42, 1995.

125. SUH, H., JUN, H.W. Effectiveness and mode of action of isopropyl myristate as a permeation enhancer for naproxen through shed snake skin. **J. *Pharm. Pharmacol*.** 48, 812- 816, 1996.

126. TAKAHASHI, K., TAMAGAWA, S., KATAGI, T., RYTTING, J.H., NISHIHATA, T., MIZUNO, N. Percutaneous penetration of basic compounds through shed snake skin as a model membrane. ***J. Pharm. Pharmacol.*** 45, 882-886, 1993.

127. TAKAHASHI, K.; SAKANO, H.; RYTTING, J.H.; NUMATA, N.; KURODA, S.;MIZUNO, N. Influence of pH on the permeability of p-toluidine and aminopyrine through shed skin as a model membrane. ***Drug Dev. Ind. Pharm.*** 27:159-164, 2001.

128. TAKAHASHI, K.; TAMAGAWA, S.; KATAGI, T.;RYTTING, J.H.; NISHIHATA, T.; MIZUNO, N. TURUNEN, T.M., BUYUKTIMKIN, S., BUYUKTIMKIN, N., URTTI, A., PARONEN, P., RYTTING, J.H. Enhanced delivery of 5-fluorouracil through shed snake skin by two new transdermal penetration enhancers**. *Int. J. Pharm*.** 92, 89-95, 1993.

129. TIOSSI R. F. J. T. ; COSTA, J. C. ; MIRANDA M.A.; PRAÇA, F.S.G. ; BENTLEY, M. V. L. B. ; BASTOS J. K. A validated HPLC analytical method for the analysis of solasonine and solamargine in in vitro skin penetration studies. ***Quimica Nova***, 35:2312-2316, 2012.

130. TREGEAR, R.T. Relative penetrability of hair follicles and epidermis. ***J. Physiology***, 156 (2):307-313, 1961.

131. TREHERNE, J.E. The permeability of skin to some non-electrolytes. ***J. Physiology***, 133(1): 171-180, 1956.

132. UNITED STATES PHARMACOPEIA: USP 31. The National Formulary: NF22. Rockville: United States Pharmacopeial Convention, 2008.

133. USP 29, UNITED STATES PHARMACOPOEIA. 29.ed. Rockville: United States Pharmacopoeial Convention, 2006.

134. WAGNER, J. G. Biopharmaceutics and Relevant Pharmacokinetics. Hamilton: ***Drug Intelligence Publications***, pg 375, 1971.

135. WIDLER N, SIGRIST A, GAFNER FM. Lipid analysis and transepidermal water loss in snakes. ***IFSCC Magazine*** v.5 (1): 24-29, 2002.

136. WILLIAMS, A.C.; BARRY, B.W. Penetration enhancers. ***Adv. Drug Delivery Rev.***, 56(5):603-618, 2004.

137. WONG, O., HUNTINGTON, J., NISHIHATA, T., RYTTING, J.H. New alkyl N,N- dialkyl-substituted amino acetates as transdermal penetration enhancers. ***Pharm. Res***. 6, 286-295, 1989.

138. WOOLLEY-HART A. A simple technique for measuring skin conductivity. ***Med Biol Eng***, 10(4):561-3, 1972.

139. ZATZ, J.L. Skin permeation. Fundamentals and application. Wheaton: Allured Publishing

Corporation, 300p, 1993.

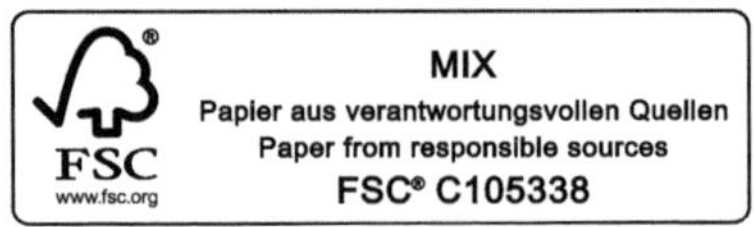

Printed by Books on Demand GmbH, Norderstedt / Germany